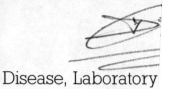

Disease, Laboratory

Disease, Laboratory Data and Diagnosis:
20 Cases to Improve Diagnostic Skills

V. Schwarz, PhD
Reader, Departments of Chemical Pathology and Child Health,
University of Manchester

G. M. Addison, MA, MB, B.Chir, PhD
Consultant Chemical Pathologist, Department of Clinical Pathology,
Royal Manchesters and Booth Hall Children's Hospital

Butterworths
London Boston Durban Singapore Sydney Toronto Wellington

First published, 1985

© **Butterworth & Co. (Publishers) Ltd, 1985**

British Library Cataloguing in Publication Data

Schwarz, V.
  Disease, laboratory data and diagnosis :
  20 cases to improve diagnostic skills.
  1. Diseases — Case studies
  I. Title   II. Addison, G. M.
  616'.09   RC66

  ISBN 0-407-00540-4

Library of Congress Cataloguing in Publication Data

Schwarz, Victor.
  Disease, laboratory data and diagnosis.

  Includes bibliographies and index.
  1. Diagnosis, Differential. 2. Diagnosis,
Laboratory. I. Addison, G. M. (Gerald Michael)
II. Title. [DNLM: 1. Diagnosis, Differential.
2. Diagnosis, Laboratory. WB 141.5 S411d]
RC71.5.S38   1985   616.07'5   84-20074
ISBN 0-407-00540-4

Photoset by Illustrated Arts Limited, Sutton, Surrey
Printed and bound in England by A. Wheaton & Co. Ltd., Exeter

Foreword

The authors in so kindly inviting me to consider contributing a foreword to this book also wondered 'whether you like the idea of case-based books'. My response was that whilst I was certainly not against them, the few that I had looked at had not greatly impressed me. After sampling this book, although not in minute detail, I can say that I am very strongly in favour of 'case-based books' – when they are written by Victor Schwarz and Michael Addison. The clinical students at Manchester are indeed blessed to have teachers of chemical pathology who offer optional evening seminars structured in this way, and I am not surprised to learn that these are popular.

The approach adopted in this book not only provides an excellent education in the use and interpretation of laboratory data but also adds a substantial amount of revision in metabolism and therapeutics. The key to the success of the whole enterprise is the placing of the information and interrogation as close as possible to actual clinical practice. Indeed these presentations could be considered as paper exercises in clinical practice.

It seems to me that to be of maximum benefit to medical students these presentations should be explored at a relatively late stage in the curriculum because they call for the integration of so much curricular information. However, one could also envisage that the early exhibition of one or two of these cases would serve to impress upon medical students something of the scope of the information which is brought to bear in the diagnosis and treatment of a single patient. I suppose it is too much to hope that the perpetual medical student question 'do we have to know . . . ?' would be silenced by a reading of this book.

At the other end of medical education people embarking on specialist training will find much of value in this material because the questions posed can be answered at different depths. One hopes too that the style and structure of the presentations will interest more senior people with specialized knowledge in debating the emphasis and interpretations provided. One of the fascinations of medicine is the variety of ways in which a particular problem can be approached.

Believing as I do that this book can be used in different ways at different stages of medical education, it is hoped that the authors will have the energy to go on to a second set of cases and that others will be motivated to undertake variations on this theme.

C. N. Hales
Professor of Clinical Biochemistry
University of Cambridge

Acknowledgements

We gratefully acknowledge the contributions made by our colleagues to the collection and discussion of cases for the departmental seminars, a few of which have formed the basis of the cases presented here: Professor J. G. Ratcliffe, Drs A. H. Gowenlock, E. Gowland and C. Weinkove, and the late Professor J. R. Daly. We would also like to thank Professor Hale for kindly agreeing to write the Foreword.

Preface

The ideas on which this book is based sprang from optional evening seminars organized for our clinical students by the Department of Chemical Pathology. Their object is to challenge the student to proceed by a logical analysis of case history, clinical examination and laboratory investigations to the differential diagnosis, a consideration of further investigations needed and the therapy indicated. The popularity of the seminars and the good record of attendance over the years persuaded us of the educational value of stimulating the learning process by the challenge of an actual case.

While the direct interaction between tutor and student is clearly superior to the printed page, we hope that our system of Leading Questions which follow each case presentation will help the reader to develop a logical approach to solving the problems faced and to improve his diagnostic skills. The 20 cases, adapted from the authors' own experience or the literature, cover a broad spectrum of diseases and the laboratory investigations pertinent to them and we feel that they constitute a valuable adjunct to perusal of textbook or lecture notes. The full discussion of each case includes material often somewhat beyond the requirements of a first degree course but which we deemed interesting and illuminating. Together with suggested further reading, our cases will also be found useful by students for higher qualifications.

We consider the main value of our presentation to be twofold: (a) it provides motivation for understanding the patient's manifestations and the significance of laboratory tests; (b) it encourages a systematic, rational approach to diagnosis and therapy. We therefore urge the reader carefully to consider each question and to write down the answer as best he can before proceeding to the next one. The Leading Questions are intended either to guide the student ultimately to the solution of the problem or to draw his attention to particularly important aspects.

The reference ranges vary somewhat as they are those in current use by the hospital laboratories that have performed the respective investigations.

V. Schwarz
G. M. Addison

Case 1

Case History

A 45-year-old man was brought by ambulance to the emergency department at 02.45 hours. He was accompanied by his wife who reported that he had been taken ill at a party, about 2 hours after a heavy meal and much drink. Within 30 minutes his abdominal pain had become so severe that they had to call a doctor who had requested his admission to hospital. The pain was in the epigastrium, was constant in intensity and radiated to his back. He had vomited several times, first the gastric contents and later a greenish fluid with much mucus. He had been well, apart from occasional bouts of 'indigestion'.

Examination

The patient was obviously in great pain and lay on his side with his knees drawn up. He was pale, sweaty and retching. There was no anaemia or jaundice but the patient was clinically moderately dehydrated with reduced skin turgor.

CVS Pulse 120 per minute regular.
      Blood pressure 110/70 mm Hg (lying).
AS   The upper abdomen was distended with epigastric tenderness on deep palpation and muscle guarding. No masses were palpated.
All other systems: no abnormality detected.
X-rays Chest X-ray: no abnormality detected.
         Abdominal X-ray: erect and supine, unremarkable.
ECG   sinus tachycardia.

Laboratory investigations

On admission

Investigation	Result	Reference range
Haemoglobin (g/dl)	13·0	13·0 – 17·0
Red blood cells ($10^{12}.\ \ell^{-1}$)	4·5	4·2 – 6·5
White blood cells ($10^9.\ \ell^{-1}$)	7·8	4 – 11
Serum sodium (mmol. ℓ^{-1})	140	135 – 145
Serum potassium (mmol. ℓ^{-1})	2·9	3·3 – 5·3
Serum urea (mmol. ℓ^{-1})	6·9	2·5 – 7·5
Blood glucose (mmol. ℓ^{-1}) (random)	8·6	3·3 – 8·4

Twelve hours later the patient's condition had deteriorated. Although his abdominal pain had lessened somewhat, it was in the same position. He was still dehydrated, he was now hyperventilating and he started passing red urine.

Further laboratory tests – 12 hours later

Investigation	Result	Reference range
Haemoglobin (g/dl)[a]	12·1	13·0 – 17·0
Serum sodium (mmol. ℓ^{-1})	141	135 – 145
Serum potassium (mmol. ℓ^{-1})	5·0	3·3 – 5·3
Serum chloride (mmol. ℓ^{-1})	105	98 – 108
Serum urea (mmol. ℓ^{-1})	11·9	2·5 – 7·5
Serum calcium (mmol. ℓ^{-1})	2·05	2·25 – 2·65
Serum creatinine (mmol. ℓ^{-1})	170	60 – 120
Blood glucose (fasting) (mmol. ℓ^{-1})	5·6	2·5 – 5·0
Total protein (g. ℓ^{-1})	55	62 – 82
Albumin (g. ℓ^{-1})	34	35 – 50
Serum amylase (IU. ℓ^{-1})	1280	75 – 260
Serum alkaline phosphatase (IU. ℓ^{-1})	98	30 – 110
Serum alanine aminotransferase (ALT) (IU. ℓ^{-1})	350	15 – 55
Serum lactic dehydrogenase (LDH) (IU. ℓ^{-1})	680	120 – 365
pH	7·25	7·32 – 7·49
P_{CO_2} (mm Hg)	21	27 – 41
P_{O_2} (mm Hg)	71	80 – 105
Bicarbonate (mmol. ℓ^{-1})	11·8	18 – 27
Base excess (mmol. ℓ^{-1})	− 10·8	−6 – 1

[a] Haemoglobinaemia now apparent.

Questions

1. What is the differential diagnosis?
2. Are there any further investigations you would request?
3. How would you treat the patient? What is the prognosis?

Leading Questions

1. (a) What tentative conclusions can be drawn from the location and the intensity of the pain, the time and nature of onset and its persistence at constant level?
   (b) The location of the pain suggests at least 15 different conditions which could give rise to it. What are they?
   (c) Are any of them unlikely in view of the history and clinical examination?

(d) Do the ECG and X-rays help in eliminating some causes?

(e) Which possible diagnosis would be associated with a much higher blood glucose?

(f) Can you account for the low serum K on admission?

(g) Which is the most informative laboratory test 12 hours later? Is it pathognomonic for a particular disease?

(h) Why is the urine red and how does this observation help to build up the picture created by other tests?

(i) A greatly raised alkaline phosphatase would have pointed strongly at one particular diagnosis. What is it?

(j) Could damage to one particular cell type account for the elevated LDH as well as another biochemical abnormality reported at 12 hours?

(k) What conclusion do you draw from the raised serum urea and creatinine and which two likely pathological processes could account for it?

(l) In the absence of any manifest pulmonary or cardiac abnormality how do you explain the mild hypoxaemia?

(m) What is the nature and cause of the acidosis?

2. (a) In the light of the diagnosis, what further tests would show the development of sequelae in the chief affected organ and possible damage to neighbouring structures?

(b) Why is the serum calcium low? Is it likely to fall further?

(c) How would you assess the extent of the renal damage?

3. (a) What are the main agents responsible for tissue damage? How can their action be curbed?

(b) Why is one particular analgesic avoided?

(c) What is the first and immediate therapeutic measure, irrespective of the diagnosis?

(d) What other measures are required to correct biochemical abnormalities?

(e) If the patient survives, what advice would you offer?

Discussion

The patient presents as an 'acute abdomen', with epigastric pain radiating to the back and vomiting. The pain is clearly severe, as judged by the patient's fetal position, and it seems to have been precipitated by a heavy meal and alcohol. It has developed quite rapidly, building up to a maximum intensity in 30 minutes and has remained constant in nature, intensity and location. The description is classical for acute pancreatitis, but a number of other acute conditions must be considered. The pain associated with a perforation strikes more suddenly, whereas a stone is more likely to give rise to an intermittent, waxing and waning colic as it moves in the biliary or urinary tract. On the other hand, the build-up to a constant intensity suggests an inflammatory condition like pancreatitis, appendicitis or diverticulitis, the first of these fitting the location of the pain better than the last two.

Notwithstanding these early impressions, consideration must be given to other possible causes of persistent pain in the epigastrium: gastritis, perforated gastric or duodenal ulcer or diverticulum, acute hepatitis or cholecystitis, pancreatitis, intestinal obstruction, appendicitis, stones in the biliary or urinary tracts, pulmonary or cardiovascular disease and finally metabolic causes such as diabetic ketoacidosis, heavy metal poisoning, acute porphyria and hypercalcaemia.

Elimination of some causes

In the absence of cough or respiratory difficulties and cardiovascular symptoms pulmonary and cardiac disease is unlikely. Acute hepatitis or cholecystitis present with pain in the upper quadrant and do not usually lead to shock, which is more in line with pancreatitis, perforated ulcer or a mesenteric catastrophe. Of these pancreatitis fits the clinical evidence best.

The clear chest X-ray and the normal ECG militate against pulmonary and cardiac disease. Perforation of the bowel would manifest itself as free air under the diaphragm: none is seen on the X-ray. A glucose level only slightly above the upper limit of normal is not consistent with diabetic ketoacidosis and is more likely to be due to sympathetic hyperactivity promoted by shock. The only other abnormal biochemical value on admission is the low serum K which may be referable to K loss in the vomitus.

Serum amylase

Of the investigations done 12 hours later the serum amylase is the most useful: it establishes pancreatitis as the primary diagnosis. It should be noted, however, that the serum amylase may be moderately raised in several acute conditions, though generally not more than 3–5 times the upper limit of the normal range, e.g., common bile duct obstruction, cholecystitis, perforated duodenal ulcer, intestinal obstruction, appendicitis, afferent loop syndrome, ketoacidosis, mesenteric ischaemia, aortic aneurysm, and others, less easily confused with pancreatitis. On the other hand, elevation of the serum amylase is often moderate and in any case transitory in pancreatitis and hence even a normal level does not rule out this diagnosis; nor does the magnitude of the rise correlate with the severity of the disease. The urine amylase persists somewhat longer and is claimed to be a more sensitive index of acute pancreatitis but it is no more diagnostic than the serum amylase.

Other enzymes and haemoglobin

The patient's haemoglobinaemia and haemoglobinuria (red urine) are indicative of intravascular haemolysis which contributes to the 0·9 g/dl fall in haemoglobin concentration and the rise in serum K. We cannot be sure about the origin of ALT: it could be derived from the pancreas itself or from some other organ damaged by poor tissue perfusion. The alkaline phosphatase is within normal limits and offers some reassurance that the inflamed pancreas has not obstructed the bile duct. LDH derives mainly from the haemolyzed red cells, although muscle ischaemia may have contributed. Renal damage, either due to inadequate perfusion or the haemoglobinaemia, is indicated by the elevated urea and creatinine.

The mild hypoxaemia is almost certainly due to inadequate ventilation caused by abdominal distention impairing the movement of the diaphragm, and possibly to surfactant being degraded by pancreatic phospholipase A. The low pH, bicarbonate and negative base excess indicate a metabolic acidosis, partly compensated by respiratory alkalosis, which may be the consequence of poor tissue perfusion or of release of H^+ from cells destroyed by autodigestion.

Further tests

The diagnosis of pancreatitis should be supplemented by ultrasonic investigation of the biliary system and of the pancreas itself for pseudocysts; a determination of serum bilirubin and urine urobilinogen to indicate any blockage of the bile duct, repeat determinations of calcium which is at the lower end of the normal range and liable to fall further. Hypocalcaemia in pancreatitis has long been ascribed to sequestration as calcium soap following hydrolysis of triglycerides, but a partial failure of the homeostatic regulation involving parathyroid hormone seems at least as likely. The extent and progress of tubular damage must be kept under review by estimation of urine volume and concentration. Blood glucose must be monitored to detect any damage to the endocrine pancreas.

Pathogenesis

Ideally the treatment of pancreatitis would be to protect the organ itself and the surrounding tissues from the damaging effects of escaping active pancreatic enzymes. The pathogenesis of the disease is generally accepted to be based on autodigestion, even if the triggering mechanism is still unclear and possibly dependent on the aetiology. Alcohol abuse seems to have a toxic effect on the pancreas as it does on the liver, and ischaemia or excessive stimulation by CCK-PZ or vagal activity also may sensitize the gland. In that state the organ is apparently unable to resist the onslaught by regurgitated duodenal contents with their highly active mixtures of proteolytic enzymes, bile acids, lysolecithin and bacteria. The protective action of endogenous protease inhibitors is overcome and the regurgitated trypsin is able to activate pancreatic trypsinogen and chymotripsinogen, thus compounding the proteolytic capability of the fluid in and around the gland. Histamine is released and the kinin system is activated, with increase in capillary permeability. A cascade of activation of other pro-enzymes causes destruction of membranes, organelles and stroma, resulting in oedema, pain, invasion by leucocytes, haemorrhage and necrosis. Liberation of lipase leads to fat necrosis, while proteolytic attack on C3 yields a leucotactic peptide which is a potent mediator of the local inflammatory response. Blood and tissue fluid proteins become substrates for the rampant proteases with formation of toxic products. Large amounts of fluid are sequestered in the retroperitoneal space, so reducing substantially the circulating blood volume.

Treatment

Little can be done to stem this disastrous sequence of events. Trasylol, a trypsin inhibitor, has never been clearly shown to be effective, nor has the putative inhibition of pancreatic enzyme secretion by glucagon been demonstrated. The treatment consists of parenteral fluid and nutrition, naso-gastric suction to minimize antral distention and release of gastrin, exchange transfusion, if necessary, to remove haemoglobin, administration of calcium gluconate to maintain an adequate calcium level and prevent tetany. Pethidine is the preferred analgesic: morphine is precluded by its action on the sphincter of Oddi. In the longterm avoidance of alcohol is mandatory.

Additional Questions

In which respects would the history, examination and laboratory investigations have differed if the patient had presented with:
1. A perforated duodenal ulcer?
2. Mesenteric artery occlusion?
3. Pulmonary embolus to the lower lobe?

Further Reading

Duerr, G. H-K. (1979) Acute Pancreatitis, in *The Exocrine Pancreas*, ed. Howat, H. T. and Sarles, H., pp. 352–393, W. B. Saunders Co. Ltd., London.
Gillespie, I. (1981), Acute Pancreatitis, *Practitioner*, **225**, pp. 463–471.

Case 2

Case History

Mrs A. L., a 32-year-old staff nurse, presented to her GP with a history of anxiety which she said had worsened since a recent promotion had increased her responsibilities. Further questioning elucidated that she slept poorly, perspired excessively, had lost a small amount of weight despite a good appetite and had noticed a slight increase in bowel habit with loosely formed motions. During her interview she continually fidgeted, was unable to sit still and at one time broke down and cried. The patient stated she was taking no drugs except for oral contraceptives.

A family history revealed that an aunt had pernicious anaemia and her sister insulin dependent diabetes mellitus.

Examination

The patient appeared anxious and was noticeably hyperkinetic. Her skin was warm and moist and she wore few clothes despite the cold weather. There was marked retraction of the upper eye lid but no exophthalmos.

CVS   Pulse 120 per minute regular.
       Blood pressure 130/60 mm Hg (lying).
       Apex beat – forceful and bounding but not displaced.

RS   Respiratory rate 28 per minute.

CNS   Fine tremor of the hands.
       Brisk reflexes.

Neck Thyroid moderately enlarged, painless, diffuse and soft.

Questions

1. What is the differential diagnosis?
2. What investigations would you do to confirm the clinical diagnosis?
3. What treatment is available and how would you monitor its effectiveness?

Leading Questions

1. (a) Do the main signs and symptoms favour one particular diagnosis?
   (b) What alternative diagnoses involving endogenous or exogenous pathophysiological or psychological factors are compatible with some of the symptoms?
2. (a) What laboratory tests should be performed to confirm or refute the most likely diagnosis?
   (b) What interpretive problems are posed by the nature of·the physiological substance(s) implicated, or the regulation of its (their) concentration and transport in plasma?
   (c) Which of the tests would you expect to be the most informative on physiological grounds?
   (d) Can drugs or variations in normal physiology influence the results, and if so, how may these variations be corrected for?
   (e) What dynamic tests are available to investigate borderline cases further?
   (f) If these tests are negative what other tests should be done to investigate alternative diagnoses?
   (g) Is the family history useful in making the diagnosis?
3. (a) What is the main objective of treatment? What alternative methods are available to achieve this objective?
   (b) What biochemical tests would best indicate the adequacy of treatment?

Discussion

The clinical diagnosis of this case is not difficult especially once the examination has been completed. However, on the basis of the history a number of diagnoses should be considered. In a patient of this age, thyrotoxicosis, anxiety states and drug abuse are the main ones. Two other rare disorders worth considering are phaeo-chromocytoma and carcinoid. In an older patient chronic obstructive bronchitis with CO_2 retention can give rise to similar symptoms. Thyrotoxicosis, anxiety states and drug abuse particularly of stimulants such as caffeine, amphetamines, cocaine and LSD have many signs and symptoms in common, including nervous irritability and lability, restlessness, palpitations, insomnia, tachycardia, hyperreflexia and increased blood pressure. Thyrotoxic and anxiety state patients both complain of fatigue, although in the former case the desire for physical activity is still present; the tachycardia of the thyrotoxic patient is present during sleep while in anxiety states the sleeping pulse is usually normal. The blood pressure elevation in thyrotoxicosis can also be distinguished by a wide pulse pressure due to the simultaneous increase in the systolic and lowering of the diastolic pressures.

Many of the symptoms of thyrotoxicosis, including lid retraction, are due to increased adrenergic activity. It is not surprising therefore that the symptoms of phaeochromocytoma are similar. The sympathomimetic symptoms are due in part to an increase in the number of beta adrenergic receptors and hence altered sensitivity to catecholamines. However, in order for this increased sensitivity to manifest itself clinically, the negative feedback control on central sympathetic outflow must also be altered.

Laboratory Tests

If the aetiology is still in doubt after the clinical examination a number of biochemical investigations will need to be performed. These are thyroid function tests, screening for drugs of abuse and urinary hydroxymethylmandelic acid (HMMA) and 5-hydroxy-indoleacetic acid (5-HIAA). In this patient the enlarged and painless goiter means that she almost certainly has thyrotoxicosis. The diagnosis can be confirmed by carrying out thyroid function tests; several are available but none are entirely satisfactory by themselves. The problems derive from a number of factors including the control mechanism of thyroid hormone secretion, the presence of thyroid hormone binding proteins in plasma, the existence of two types of thyroid hormone (thyroxine (T4) and triiodothyronine (T3)) and end organ metabolism of thyroid hormones. The most important technical and interpretive problems are caused by the binding of thyroxine to proteins in plasma.

Factors determining free T3 and T4

T4 is reversibly bound to three plasma proteins, thyroxine binding globulin (TBG), thyroxine binding prealbumin (TBPA) and albumin so that approximately 99.97 per cent of thyroxine is bound of which 75 per cent is bound to TBG. T3 is bound to TBG and albumin and 99.7 per cent is in this form. The hormonal activity of T4 and T3 resides in the 0.03 per cent and 0.3 per cent of free hormone respectively and it is alteration in the amount of free hormone which leads to the symptoms of thyroid disease. The normal physiological regulation of thyroid gland secretion by feedback inhibition of TSH release is also controlled by the level of the free thyroid hormones in plasma. Changes in their concentration can be brought about in three circumstances. The first is an increase or reduction in thyroid gland secretion due to primary thyroid disease. The second is an alteration of the absolute quantity of binding proteins, e.g., in pregnancy, treatment with oestrogens and androgens, inherited abnormalities of TBG synthesis, hepatic and renal diseases and starvation. The third is competition by other compounds such as drugs for the binding sites (*Table 2.1*). In the latter two instances the

Table 2.1 Drug effects on thyroid function tests

Drug	Effect
1. Oestrogens including oral contraceptives	Increase in plasma thyroxine binding globulins
2. Androgens	Decrease in plasma thyroxine binding globulins
3. Salicylates, phenytoin and other anticonvulsants	Competition for thyroxine binding sites
4. Phenytoin	Increase in T3 and T4 metabolism
5. Propranolol, X-ray contrast media	Decreased T4 to T3 conversion
6. Iodide, propylthiouracil, carbimazole	Inhibition of T3 and T4 synthesis

physiological control mechanisms will ultimately ensure a normal free hormone level and the main effects will be observed on the total (free + bound) T3 and T4.

Problems of Technique

The older biochemical methods for T4 and T3 measured the total hormone concentration in the plasma which led to errors in diagnosis in cases with more or less hormone bound to plasma proteins. A number of T3 resin binding tests were then developed which indirectly estimated the degree of saturation of the TBG. Using these tests and the total T4, a 'Free Thyroxine Index' (FTI) could be derived giving an indirect estimation of the free T4. It also became possible to measure TBG routinely by immunochemical methods and to obtain reference ranges for T4 at each level of TBG. Problems still occur, however, in patients taking drugs which compete for the hormone binding sites on the plasma proteins. More recently still a number of sensitive techniques have been developed which allow the direct determination of free T4 on a routine basis. Unfortunately even with these tests there are problems with standardization as a consequence of which the respective tests may give different results particularly in patients with moderate and severe abnormalities of TBG.

This patient is on oral contraceptives and hence her TBG, total T3 and T4 will be raised. An FTI or free T4 estimation will therefore be required to establish whether there is an abnormality of thyroid gland activity. A similar situation would occur in pregnancy. Women taking oral contraceptives constitute the largest group of patients with thyroid function tests altered by drugs; patients on chronic anticonvulsant therapy the next most common group.

In thyrotoxicosis the pattern of thyroid hormone activity varies. Most frequently both T4 and T3 are elevated but T3 alone may be elevated in some patients (T3 toxicosis). This latter finding may be transient, with T4 rising later in the course of the disease. Occasionally only T4 is elevated especially in the elderly or sick patient where T4 to T3 conversion is reduced. It is, therefore, necessary to measure both T4 and T3, together with a direct or indirect estimation of the binding proteins.

Borderline Cases

In a small number of patients inconclusive clinical and biochemical findings make diagnosis difficult. In these patients a thyrotrophin releasing hormone (TRH) test should be carried out. Plasma TSH is determined before and after IV administration of TRH: a failure to rise owing to strong feedback inhibition by circulating T4 or T3 indicates thyrotoxicosis. Again it should be noted that certain drugs affect basal TSH and the TSH response to TRH.

Aetiology

Having diagnosed thyrotoxicosis, the final stage is to establish which type. The presence of a goitre limits the cause to primary thyroid disease, in particular Graves' disease, toxic adenoma and toxic multinodular goitre. These conditions can be differentiated clinically and by thyroid scintography. Graves' disease is caused by autoantibodies which react with the TSH receptor or cell surface antigens close by on the thyroid cell. As a result adenylate cyclase is activated and the cell stimulated into synthesising and releasing thyroid hormones. These autoantibodies which so far have all been identified as IgG molecules, are collectively termed thyroid stimulating immunoglobulins (TSI) of which the best known is LATS – long acting thyroid stimulator. TSIs have been found in 95 per cent of patients with Graves' disease at some stage of their disease; levels do, however, fluctuate. Routine measurement of TSI is not generally available and their presence does not necessarily confirm the diagnosis of Graves' disease since they have been found in the serum of patients with some other thyroid disorders.

There is often a strong familial tendency in Graves' disease together with other autoimmune diseases such as pernicious anaemia. Graves' disease is associated with HLA types B8, DW3 and CW in caucasians and HLA-BW35 in Japanese.

Therapy

Treatment of Graves' disease consists of the use of antithyroid drugs, e.g., propylthiouracil and carbimazole, which inhibit thyroid hormone synthesis. Results of treatment can be judged clinically but measurement of T4 and T3 may be useful and an increase in TSH would indicate overtreatment. Adrenergic antagonists, e.g., propranolol, are useful in patients in whom the symptoms of sympathetic overactivity are excessive or in whom there is a danger of heart failure. Patients who do not respond to medical therapy or who relapse on withdrawal of treatment require surgery or radioiodine ablation of the thyroid gland.

14

Additional Questions

1. Do the various biochemical tests including measurement of TSI and HLA type assist in determining prognosis?
2. What is the main complication of treatment? How may this be avoided?

Further Reading

Hall, R. H. (1981) Thyrotrophin receptor antibodies and Graves' disease, *Hospital Update* **7**, pp. 161–172.
Wenzel, K. W. (1981). Pharmacological interference with in vitro tests of thyroid function, *Metabolism,* **30**, pp. 717–732.

Case 3

Case History

J. F., a 53-year-old ex-mill worker was admitted as an emergency. Several years previously he had taken early retirement after a prolonged history of increasing respiratory symptoms; cough with white sputum and shortness of breath. Over the last few months the shortness of breath was such that he was unable to leave his home. Two days before admission he deteriorated markedly and began to produce copious amounts of green/yellow sputum. The general practitioner found him to be semicomatose. A history of heavy smoking was obtained from the patient's wife.

Examination

The patient appeared drowsy, very depressed and confused. He was sweating and showed evidence of central cyanosis.

CVS   Pulse 120 per minute, regular.
      Blood pressure 190/120 mmHg (lying)
      JVP raised 9 cm.
      Liver enlarged.
      Gross oedema of both ankles.
      Heart: apex impalpable, sounds normal.
RS   Respiratory rate increased.
      Diminished chest movements.
      No clubbing.
      Auscultation revealed diffuse wheezing over all the chest with some crepitations at the bases.
CNS   No localizing signs.

Laboratory Investigations

Investigation	On admission	After 24% O_2	Reference range
Arterial pH	7·22	7·10	7·36–7·44
Arterial Po_2 (mm Hg)	42	49	80–105
Arterial Pco_2 (mm Hg)	67	84	35–47
Base excess (mmol. ℓ^{-1})	−4	−10	±3
Actual HCO_3 (mmol. ℓ^{-1})	27	25	22–30

Continued on next page

Laboratory Investigations contd

Investigation	On admission	Reference range
Plasma sodium (mmol. ℓ^{-1})	141	135–145
Plasma potassium (mmol. ℓ^{-1})	4·9	3·5–5·5
Plasma chloride (mmol. ℓ^{-1})	102	98–108
Plasma urea (mmol. ℓ^{-1})	5·4	2·5–7·5
Blood glucose (mmol. ℓ^{-1}) (random)	7·3	3·5–10
Haemoglobin (g. dl^{-1})	18·8	13–17
PCV (1. ℓ^{-1})	0·59	0·40–0·49
WBC ($\times 10^9$. ℓ^{-1}]	12·5	4–10

To convert Po_2, Pco_2 and reference ranges to kPa divide by 7·5.

Questions

1. What is the diagnosis?
2. Why did the treatment worsen the patient's acid base status?
3. What treatment would you prescibe and how would you monitor its effect?

Leading Questions

1. (a) There are two aspects of the case history, what are they?
   (b) Does the patient's history indicate the precipitating cause of his present condition and hence suggest appropriate laboratory investigations?
   (c) What primary diseases of the lung or of other organs could account for the patient's history and symptoms?
   (d) Do the patient's heavy smoking and occupational background favour one diagnosis?
   (e) Is there any evidence that the heart is implicated?
   (f) Is there any biochemical or haematological evidence of a chronic condition and/or a recent exacerbation?
   (g) To what extent do the results of the clinical examination reflect the disorder of function indicated by the initial laboratory investigations?
   (h) Are any further tests required to establish the diagnosis?
2. (a) Is the aggravation of the acidosis due to a metabolic or respiratory cause?
   (b) What are the normal mechanisms for controlling the acid base status?

   (c) Why has there been no change in the plasma bicarbonate despite the change in pH?

   (d) What is the mechanism of respiratory control?

   (e) What are the stimuli for this mechanism?

   (f) Are they equally potent in all circumstances?

3. (a) What is the immediate objective of treatment?

   (b) What alternatives are there if primary treatment fails?

   (c) Would treatment with bicarbonate be helpful? What are its possible disadvantages?

   (d) What is the purpose of treating the heart condition?

   (e) What long-term treatment or advice should be given?

Discussion

The clinical presentation of this patient would indicate that he has respiratory failure which, from the history, has been present for some time. The findings of the clinical examination confirm the presence of hypoxia (central cyanosis) and hypercapnia (confusion, tachycardia, sweating and hypertension from generalized sympathetic activity). Respiratory failure can be caused by diseases which interfere with ventilation alone, give rise to alterations in the ventilation-perfusion ratio in the lungs or both. Causes include primary lung disease but also diseases of other organs, e.g., heart, muscle and CNS which have secondary effects on respiration.

The production of large amounts of green/yellow sputum by this patient, coupled with the rapid deterioration, history of heavy smoking and his previous occupation suggest that the most likely diagnosis is an acute infective exacerbation of chronic obstructive bronchitis (often referred to as chronic obstructive airways disease or COAD). Respiratory disease is associated with several occupations in which the working environment is dusty. There are a number of specific disorders but the end stage is often chronic obstructive bronchitis. Other diagnoses such as chronic heart disease and carcinoma of the lung cannot be ruled out on the available information. The findings of raised JVP, enlarged liver and peripheral oedema indicate right-sided heart failure which in combination with generalized lung disease is termed 'cor pulmonale'.

Metabolic Derangements

The initial biochemical investigation confirms the presence of hypoxia and hypercapnia. Hypoxia has been present for a considerable time since the patient has polycythaemia, a hallmark of chronic hypoxia. Polycythaemia, which is an increased red cell mass, may be masked by a proportionate increase in plasma volume. Chronic hypoxia would support chronic obstructive bronchitis as the most likely diagnosis. On the other hand the hypercapnia is probably of very recent origin since there is no evidence of renal compensation of the severe respiratory acidosis. The homeostatic mechanism in the kidney for the correction of acid base disturbances involves several different processes which result in the excretion of hydrogen ion and the reabsorption of bicarbonate and sodium. A healthy kidney can compensate for changes in blood pH due to alterations in $P\mathrm{CO_2}$ but the changes are slow and take 3–5 days to restore the pH to normal.

In the present case full compensation to pH 7·4 would have required the plasma bicarbonate to rise to 40.1 mmol. ℓ^{-1}. This can be derived from the Hendersen–Hasselbalch equation itself a derivative of the law of mass action:

$$pH = pK' + \log \frac{[HCO_3']}{[H_2CO_3]}$$

If fully compensated

$$7·4 = 6·1 + \log \frac{[HCO_3']}{62 \times 0·03}$$

since $[H_2CO_3] = P_{CO_2} \times$ solubility coefficient of CO_2 in blood (0·03 mmol. ℓ^{-1}. mm Hg^{-1})

$$1·3 = \log [HCO_3'] - \log 2·01$$
$$\log [HCO_3'] = 1·3 + 0·302$$
$$[HCO_3'] = 40·1 \text{ mmol. } \ell^{-1}$$

A similar calculation can be made in SI units in which case the value of the solubility coefficient of CO_2 in blood is 0.225 (mol. ℓ^{-1}. kPa^{-1}). Since the actual bicarbonate is 27 mmol. ℓ^{-1} and the base excess (defined as the amount of strong acid required to titrate the blood to pH 7·4 at a P_{CO_2} of 40 mm Hg at 37 °C) is -3 mol. ℓ^{-1}, the renal homeostatic mechanism has not had time to work. The renal metabolic compensation of respiratory acidosis is usually only partial so that the actual bicarbonate would be somewhere between the measured value and the calculated value at pH 7·4. Alternatively, it is possible that the renal compensation has been masked by a coexisting metabolic acidosis caused by an accumulation of lactic acid as a consequence of tissue hypoxia or by the loss of base, usually bicarbonate, in renal or gastrointestinal disease. A significant concentration of lactate in plasma would manifest itself in increases in the base excess and anion gap, the difference in the plasma between the major cations sodium and potassium and the major anions chloride and bicarbonate. In a normal patient the anion gap is less than 18 mmol. ℓ^{-1} and in this patient the value is 17 mmol. ℓ^{-1}. (Some authors neglect the potassium ion when calculating the anion gap: this gives values approximately 4 mmol. ℓ^{-1} lower than the method described here.) The normal anion gap makes the presence of a lactic acidosis unlikely, while the normal urea, glucose and absence of gastrointestinal symptoms eliminate the other major causes of metabolic acidosis.

Respiratory Control

The control of respiration is highly complex, involving central rhythm generating mechanisms in the medulla, chemoreceptors in the carotid body and brain stem, various receptors in the lung and proprioceptive control of the muscles involved in breathing. In chronic obstructive bronchitis the dominant control of respiration is through the chemoreceptors brought about by the hypoxia and hypercapnia. Chronic hypoxia has a negligible effect on ventilation until the arterial blood PO_2 is less than 60 mmHg (8 kPa). In some patients with chronic lung disease and persistently raised PCO_2 the sensitivity to changes in PCO_2 is reduced. These patients are relatively poorly oxygenated, but not excessively dyspnœic and are termed 'blue bloaters'. Other patients retain sensitivity to arterial PCO_2 and remain relatively well oxygenated. To do this they have to increase respiratory work, hence they are called 'pink puffers'. The reason why the response to high PCO_2 is variable in different patients is not clearly understood but it is important when considering therapy.

The principal stimulus to respiration in chronic obstructive bronchitis is hypoxia and therapy in acute exacerbations nearly always involves the administration of oxygen. The dangers of oxygen therapy are well illustrated in this patient when an increase of inspired oxygen concentration from 21 per cent in air to 24 per cent has had a profound effect leading to a worsening of his clinical state and a rise in PCO_2 and increasing acidosis. Because of the acidosis and the increased PCO_2 the sigmoidal oxyhaemoglobin dissociation curve is shifted to the right, i.e. the haemoglobin has a lower affinity for oxygen. Whereas less oxyhaemoglobin is formed in the alveolus, its dissociation in the tissues is more complete. On balance the acidotic patient may get more or less oxygen delivered to the tissues according to the relative PO_2 values in the alveoli and tissues (*Figure 3.1*). Other factors including increased 2–3 DPG concentrations in the erythrocytes and raised PCO_2 will shift the curve further to the right. However, even at the lower pH, a 3 per cent increase in inspired oxygen will cause a rise of 15 per cent in the amount of oxyhaemoglobin formed – enough to reduce the hypoxic drive. An additional factor is operating in this patient who is a heavy smoker, such individuals having up to 15 per cent carboxyhaemoglobin, which will affect not only the oxygen saturation of the blood but also the shape of the oxyhaemoglobin dissociation curve.

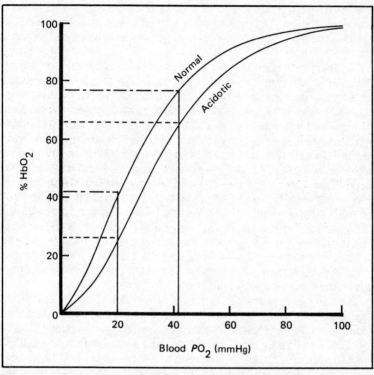

Figure 3.1 Oxyhaemoglobin dissociation curves in the normal and acidotic (pH 7·2) states showing decreased affinity of haemoglobin for oxygen at an alveolar P_{O_2} of 42 mm Hg and an increased overall oxygen release at an assumed venous P_{O_2} of 20 mm Hg. It will be seen that the effect of a shift of the curve to the right on oxygen delivery to the tissues at a lower blood pH depends in individual patients on the actual P_{O_2} values in arterial and venous blood. Total oxygen delivery to the tissues also depends on blood flow

Therapy

All these factors make the response of the individual patient to oxygen therapy difficult to predict. Oxygen therapy is therefore empirical and must be closely monitored with clinical observation and blood gas measurement. In general oxygen should not be required if the arterial P_{O_2} is greater than 60 mm Hg (8 kPa) in the absence of central cyanosis. If oxygen is given the initial concentration is governed by the P_{CO_2}. If the P_{CO_2} <50 mm Hg (6·7 kPa), 28 per cent oxygen can be given immediately but if the PCO_2 >50 mm Hg (6·7 kPa) then 24 per cent oxygen should be used and the patient's response assessed. Patients in whom large areas of the lungs are not perfused may require even higher oxygen concentrations.

Other aspects of treatment are as urgent as oxygen therapy. It is of paramount importance to clear the airways to allow maximum access for the inspired oxygen. This is achieved by frequent physiotherapy including postural drainage with chest percussion. Appropriate antibiotics must also be prescribed. If these measures fail, bronchial lavage or tracheostomy with intermittent positive pressure ventilation may rarely be required. Respiratory stimulants are of no benefit in the treatment of chronic obstructive bronchitis; some drugs including nikethamide, salicylates and theophylline may even worsen the patient's condition. Bronchodilator drugs can be used, of which salbutamol is the most suitable since it causes less tachycardia. Correction of the respiratory acidosis with sodium bicarbonate is not usually necessary and will reduce the respiratory drive from the high PCO_2 and reverse any beneficial effects of the original reduction in oxygen affinity by shifting the oxyhaemaglobin dissociation curve back to the left.

The cardiac manifestations must be treated since increasing the oxygen carrying capacity of the blood is not of much use unless the blood is being delivered to the tissues in adequate amounts. Treatment of hypoxia may even reduce the cardiac output thus cancelling the benefits of increased saturation of the haemoglobin. Diuretics may improve cor pulmonale but unwanted effects can include potassium loss and hence metabolic alkalosis which will result in a decreased response to high PCO_2 and also increases the risk of cardiac arrhythmias. Digitalis is not normally required but should be used if there is evidence of a fall in the cardiac output.

Long term management of this patient must include advice and help on giving up smoking. Changes in social conditions, employment etc. may be desirable but are difficult to achieve.

Additional Questions

1. Explain the increase in the base excess following oxygen therapy.
2. What effects does carbon monoxide have on oxygen transport and release by haemoglobin?

Further Reading

Cumming, G. and Semple, E. A. (1980). *Disorders of the Respiratory System*, 2nd edn., pp. 278–308, Blackwell Scientific Publications, Oxford.
Natelson, S. and Natelson, E. A. (1975). Maintenance of fluid and electrolyte balance, *Principles of Applied Clinical Chemistry* Vol. 1, pp. 31–36, Plenum Press, New York.

Case 4

Case History

P. F., a 46-year-old male executive, was admitted for investigation of a painful, swollen left ankle. The patient reported having attended a celebratory business function the previous evening when much food and wine had been consumed. In the early morning he had awakened with an excruciating pain in his ankle, for the relief of which he had taken six aspirins. There was no history of genito-urinary infection.

Examination

The patient was sweating and had a pyrexia of 38.2 °C. His ankle joint was swollen and red; it felt hot to the touch and was exquisitely tender and stiff so that the patient could stand only with extreme difficulty. No other joints were involved and there was no lymphadenopathy. All other systems: no abnormality detected.

Laboratory investigations

Investigation	Result	Reference range
RBC ($10^{12}.\ell^{-1}$)	5	4·2–6·5
WBC ($10^9.\ell^{-1}$)	14	4·0–11·0
Differential count	85% PMN	
Blood glucose (fasting), (mmol. ℓ^{-1})	6·8	3·0–5·3
Serum urea, (mmol. ℓ^{-1})	7·5	2·5–7·5
Serum uric acid, (μmol. ℓ^{-1})	400	245–530
(mg/dl)	6·7	4·1–8·9
Urine volume, (ml/24h)	1200	
Urine uric acid, (mmol/24h)	4·8	1·2–3·0
(g/24h)	0·8	0·2–0·5
Urine pH	6·2	4·5–7·8

Synovial fluid aspirated from ankle joint:
Cloudy, yellowish, aseptic.
White blood cells $25 \times 10^9. \ell^{-1}$
Glucose, (mmol. ℓ^{-1})　4·2　(fluid/serum glucose = 0·62)
Polarized light microscopy shows birefringent needle-shaped crystals, both free in the fluid and inside leukocytes

Questions

1. What is the differential diagnosis?
2. What is the pathogenesis and aetiology of the condition?
3. How should it be treated?

Leading Questions

1. (a) Which diagnosis is the most likely from the case history alone?
   (b) What other conditions may present somewhat similarly?
   (c) Which of the alternative diagnoses are unlikely in view of:
      (i) the absence of infection,
      (ii) the absence of lymphadenopathy,
      (iii) the absence of skin eruptions and of cardiac involvement,
      (iv) the nature of the pain,
      (v) the sudden onset of the pain and its unilateral occurrence?
   (d) Which laboratory investigation is diagnostically the most definitive in this patient?
   (e) What are the crystals found in the synovial fluid?
2. (a) The solubility of monosodium urate is influenced by a number of factors. What are they?
   (b) Why do urate crystals (and certain other crystals) cause gouty arthritis when sodium urate in solution is harmless?
   (c) How does the kidney handle uric acid and how is this affected by acids, corticosteroids or drugs?
   (d) How does the urine pH affect the solubility of monosodium urate?
   (e) Might you expect to find kidney damage in this condition? Is there any evidence for it?
   (f) If under-secretion of urate can be ruled out, to what can the hyperuricaemia be ascribed which must have preceded the precipitation of crystals?
   (g) Why do you think the blood glucose is raised? Does this offer a possible explanation for the patient's serum urate being within the normal range?
3. (a) What is the immediate aim of therapy after an attack?
   (b) Given that hyperuricaemia is a precondition for the development of gouty arthritis, at which points can this problem be tackled?
   (c) Are dietary measures helpful?

Discussion

A middle-aged business executive develops a sudden sharp pain in a peripheral joint after an eating and drinking bout. The single affected joint is inflamed, hot and swollen. These are 'classic' circumstances in an attack of gout, although in many cases alcohol is not involved. The patient's throat is not sore, there is no evidence of any other infectious foci and he has been well until now. Thus the pyrexia may reflect the inflammatory response itself rather than an infection, although the raised WBC and the leukocytes in the urine are compatible with either possibility.

The differential diagnosis includes pseudogout, Reiter's syndrome, other causes of arthritis, cellulitis, bursitis, tendonitis, thrombophlebitis and acute rheumatic fever, as well as gout. In the absence of lymphadenopathy and genito-urinary tract infection, septic arthritis or cellulitis are unlikely, while rheumatic fever usually follows an infection of the upper respiratory tract and is accompanied by skin eruptions or cardiac involvement. Thrombophlebitis is characterized by more generalized swelling and is much less painful. In acute bursitis the swelling is limited to the bursa and the distended sac is easily palpated. Rheumatoid arthritis has a much more insidious onset and usually a symmetrical involvement.

Hyperuricaemia in diagnosis

An attack of gout must be preceded by hyperuricaemia and supersaturation of ECF for crystallization of urate to occur. Thus the diagnosis of the condition is often based on the demonstration of an elevated serum urate concentration. However, definition of hyperuricaemia depends on the population examined as well as the laboratory method employed. Also, the rise in serum urate may be intermittent and therefore missed, or it may be relatively shortlived because of the uricosuric action of corticosteroids which are liable to be secreted in response to the stress of a gouty attack. In this patient the slightly elevated fasting glucose suggests that increased cortisol secretion may indeed have contributed to a lowering of the serum urate and a concomitant raising of the urinary urate. Yet the latter is within normal limits, which may reflect a modest dietary intake of purines and a normal endogenous production. Thus the present case demonstrates that the basic laboratory tests for gout may, on occasion, be negative. Even when the serum urate is raised, often in the range 420–720 μmol. ℓ^{-1} (7–12 mg/dl), the extent of the rise is not necessarily related to the severity of the attack.

It is the nature of the synovial fluid obtained from the affected ankle which provides the definitive evidence in this case. The fluid contained large numbers of leukocytes and is thus clearly inflammatory; it is aseptic and the fluid/plasma glucose ratio is relatively high, so excluding bacterial infection of the joint as a cause of the inflammation. The birefringence and needle-shape readily identifies the crystals as monosodium urate and excludes pseudogout caused by precipitation of calcium pyrophosphate. Thus we have a fairly typical case of gout.

Solubility and precipitation

Several factors contribute to the crystallization of urate in a particular site. The solubility of monosodium urate in 0·13 molar saline at 37 °C is 400 μmol. ℓ^{-1} (6·8 mg/dl), but it is increased slightly by plasma proteins. However, stable supersaturated solutions up to 14 times that concentration have been found in patients. As would be expected, the solubility is rather less at lower temperatures, being only 270 μmol. ℓ^{-1} (4·5 mg/dl) at 30 °C, and it is therefore possible for crystallization to take place in an ankle joint at its normal temperature of 29 °C when it occurs nowhere else. Proteoglycans, hyaluronic acid and chondroitin sulphate in synovial fluid are believed to increase the solubility of urate and hence conditions involving changes in structure, concentration or metabolism of these components may predispose to precipitation. The big toe, which is subjected to disproportionate stress and hence is particularly prone to degenerative changes, is often the first joint attacked and is ultimately affected in 90 per cent of patients with gout. Yet another factor bearing on the crystallization of urate in damaged joints may be the reabsorption of fluids from traumatic effusions during the night: since water clears the membranes more rapidly than urate, the concentration of the salt in the synovial fluid will rise and cause precipitation in the early morning; this is the time when gouty attacks occur most frequently. Tophaceous deposits of urate crystals may form also in other cartilagenous sites such as ear lobes and will redissolve only when the uric acid concentration in the ECF falls below 415 μmol. ℓ^{-1} (7 mg/dl). They are pathognomonic for the disease.

Inflammatory response to crystals

The mechanism by which urate crystals induce an acute inflammatory response is not completely understood. When ingested by leukocyte phagosomes they disrupt the membrane and cause hydrolytic enzymes to spill into the cytoplasm and ultimately into the synovial fluid. Silica and calcium pyrophosphate crystals act similarly. It is interesting to note in this context that lysosomal membranes containing testosterone are more prone to be ruptured by crystals, whereas membranes containing oestradiol are more resistent. This observation may well account for men and menopausal women being the main sufferers from gout. Chemotactic factor liberated from ruptured lysosomes attracts PMN leukocytes which complete the digestion of collagen fibrils and proteoglycan aggregates initiated by free collagenase and proteinases, ultimately leading to the destruction of the joint typical of the arthritic process.

Renal handling or urate

Being a small molecule, uric acid passes readily through membranes and filters freely at the glomerulus, to be reabsorbed and re-secreted at various levels of the proximal and distal tubules. Thus excretion in the urine is a function of tubular transport in both directions, ranging from 1·8–3·0 mmol/24 hours (300–500 mg/24 hours) on a low purine diet, to 600–700 mg on an average diet and up to 1 g daily on a high meat intake.

Acids in general depress excretion of uric acid and thus the ketoacidosis associated with uncontrolled diabetes or starvation and the lactic acidosis following prolonged exercise or alcohol ingestion are hyperuricaemic. Presumably this is the reason for precipitation of urate crystals in the patient. In view of the complexity of renal handling it is not surprising that many drugs interfere with one process or ·the other: some impair tubular secretion, e.g., small doses of salicylates or thiazide diuretics, and so raise the serum concentration; others stimulate excretion and hence lower the serum concentration, e.g., probenecid and larger doses of salicylates. The latter may have contributed to the patient's normal serum urate.

Failure to neutralize an acid urine above pH 6·0 is liable to result in precipitation of free uric acid in the tubular fluid and hence in formation of stones, gravel or sludge, often before the onset of arthritis. The stones are radiolucent if they consist only of uric acid but they can be seen on X-rays if they contain calcium oxalate or phosphate. For reasons not altogether clear, inadequate renal production of ammonia is not uncommon in gout and contributes to the excretion of acidic urine. In gout of longer standing renal disease is a common sequela, with mild albuminuria, benign hypertension and moderate nitrogen retention.

Overproduction

As well as under-excretion, overproduction of uric acid can lead to hyperuricaemia. The excess purine may be the result of an inborn enzyme defect, such as deficiency of hypoxanthine-guanine phos-phoryltransferase of the Lesch-Nyhan syndrome, or of an increased cellular turnover associated with proliferative disorders, e.g., polycythaemia, leukaemia, pernicious anaemia, chronic haemolytic anaemia and psoriasis. Alternatively, it may be of exogenous origin due to excess consumption of meat, which, together with over-indulgence in alcohol is well known to account for the high inci-dence of gout in the well-to-do. It seems likely that this patient's single attack was caused by the combination of high meat and alcohol intake. His renal function is normal, as indicated by the serum urea, and with a urine pH of 6·2 the kidney is well able to excrete the extra uric acid responsible for the episode of hyperuricaemia, rapidly ended by the uricosuric effects of cortisol and aspirin.

Treatment

The aim of therapy is twofold: First, to terminate the acute attack with an anti-inflammatory drug or, alternatively, to limit leukocyte activity by means of the long-established but still useful colchicine which is believed to stabilize lysosomes and curb leukocyte migra-tion. This action has diagnostic significance in so far as a beneficial effect in the early phase of the attack strongly supports the diagnosis of gout. In the longer term, colchicine can be used prophylactically to prevent leukocyte participation in the pathogenetic process. Second, if the serum uric acid concentration is above the normal limit or if there are repeated attacks or tophaceous deposits, the aim is to aid excretion by the use of uricosuric drugs, e.g., probenecid. Evaluation of uric acid production by measuring the 24 hour urine excretion while the patient is on low purine diet should indicate whether the attack was provoked by endogenous overproduction or excessive intake. The uricosuric drugs increase renal clearance of uric acid and their use has greatly improved longterm therapy and prognosis. In overproducers with a history of urinary calculi or elevated serum urate on the maximum tolerated dose of uricosuric drug, allopurinol is particularly useful. It inhibits xanthine oxidase and so stops metabolism at hypoxanthine which has a higher renal clearance than uric acid; in addition, the drug is readily converted into the corresponding ribonucleotide which inhibits the rate-limiting enzyme in purine biosynthesis.

Other therapeutic measures which contribute to or even substitute for drug treatment are high fluid intake, alkalinization of the urine with sodium bicarbonate or citrate, reduced meat intake, low fat diet (to prevent ketonuria) and avoidance of alcohol.

Additional Questions

1. Is extra-renal disposal of urate significant in:
    (a) healthy individuals
    (b) patients with renal failure?
2. What is gouty nephropathy? Why is monosodium urate particularly liable to be deposited in the renal medulla?

Further Reading

Boss, G. R. and Seegmiller, J. E. (1979) Hyperuricaemia and gout, *New Engl. J. Med.*, **300**, pp. 1459–66.

Case 5

Case History

A 21-year-old woman was seen in the outpatients department for investigation of irregular menses. One year previously she had had an appendectomy after which she remained in hospital for 3 weeks as the wound was slow in healing. A few months later she consulted her general practitioner with symptoms of weakness, severe depression and weight gain. She admitted on questioning that bruises appeared for no known reason.

Examination

The patient had truncal and facial obesity. There was acne on her face and bruising on the legs and arms.
CVS   Pulse 80 per minute regular.
        Blood pressure 150/95 mmHg (lying).
        Heart normal.
All other systems: no abnormality detected.
X-ray of the spine and long bones were suggestive of osteoporosis, while those of the skull and abdomen were normal.

Laboratory Investigations

Investigation	Result	Reference range
Blood glucose (mmol. ℓ^{-1}) (fasting)	8·2	3·0 – 5·3
Serum sodium, (mmol. ℓ^{-1})	145	135 – 146
Serum potassium (mmol. ℓ^{-1})	3·5	3·5 – 5·1
Serum urea (mmol. ℓ^{-1})	8·3	3·7 – 8·0
Urine glucose (random specimen)	+	nil
Urine cortisol (nmol/24h)	1025	< 275

Questions

1. What is the diagnosis and how may it be confirmed on an outpatient basis?
2. What further tests are most useful for elucidating the aetiology?
3. What treatment would be appropriate to each aetiology?

Leading Questions

1. (a) Does the urinary cortisol excretion accord with the signs and symptoms?
   (b) How could feedback regulation be used to confirm the presumptive diagnosis?
   (c) What is the normal response to hypoglycaemic stress and how could a test for Cushing's syndrome be based on it?
   (d) What evidence may be obtained from plasma cortisol levels at different times of the day?
2. (a) Overproduction of cortisol arises in one of two ways. What are they?
   (b) In what circumstances is adrenocorticotrophin (ACTH) secreted in excessive amounts?
   (c) Is ACTH secretion from all sources subject to similar regulatory mechanisms?
   (d) Does the clinical presentation differ according to the source or amount of ACTH?
   (e) What is the most direct way of assessing hypersecretion of ACTH?
   (f) What would you infer from an absence of ACTH from the patient's plasma and what from:
      (i) modestly raised plasma concentration
      (ii) greatly raised plasma concentration?
   (g) Metyrapone, given in large doses over 24 hours, inhibits adrenal 11-hydroxylase. How does this drug affect pituitary output of ACTH and in which aetiology of Cushing's syndrome will this effect manifest itself as an increased 17-oxogenic steroid output compared with predrug excretion?
   (h) By what means could an adrenal neoplasm be visualized?
   (i) The ectopic ACTH syndrome can often present with sequelae of massive ACTH secretion. What are they?
   (j) What other investigations are helpful in establishing the presence of tumours?
3. (a) What is the treatment of choice of Cushing's syndrome of adrenal origin if the tumour is:
      (i) unilateral and palpable through the abdominal wall
      (ii) not detectable by any diagnostic tests? What further therapy is required after such treatment?

(b) A space-occupying pituitary tumour is unusual as a cause of Cushing's disease. What is the most common pathological lesion and what options are open in the treatment?

(c) How would you treat a patient with an inoperable ACTH-producing ectopic tumour?

Discussion

Potential diagnoses such as hypothyroidism, obesity, chronic alcoholism and depression can be quickly dismissed in view of the young woman's many manifestations characteristic of Cushing's syndrome: truncal and facial obesity owing to deposition of fat at these charateristic sites, muscular weakness, poor wound healing, easy bruising and osteoporosis due to loss of protein; mild hypertension caused by sodium retention mediated by the mineralocorticoid activity of large amounts of cortisol; menstrual disturbances and acne due to excessive androgen secretion; and hyperglycaemia, glucosuria and raised serum urea and the implied breakdown of proteins reflecting increased gluconeogenesis and impaired glucose utilisation. Iatrogenic hypercortisolism must be considered, but the polycystic ovary syndrome can be excluded on the basis of the patient's excessive cortisol excretion.

Screening tests

The 24 hour urine cortisol, here found to be well in excess of the normal level, is one of three screening tests for Cushing's syndrome, of whatever cause, which can readily be performed on day-patients without an overnight admission. The other two are the low dose dexamethasone suppression and the insulin tolerance tests. Dexamethasone is a potent synthetic glucocorticoid which acts like cortisol in the feedback regulation of corticosteroid secretion. If, after a single midnight dose of 2 mg, it suppresses cortisol output to less than 170 nmol.ℓ^{-1} plasma (6 μg/100 ml), which is the lower normal limit at 09.00 hours, Cushing's syndrome is ruled out, irrespective of the aetiology.

The insulin tolerance test is based on the fact that profound hypoglycaemia normally elicits a stress response from the higher centres and the hypothalamic-pituitary system, which raises the plasma cortisol by at least 220 nmol.ℓ^{-1} (8 μg/100 ml). An inappropriately elevated cortisol level suppresses the response, which makes this test useful in the diagnosis of even mild cases of Cushing's syndrome. Since it is not without danger, especially in children, the test is usually reserved for cases which cannot be resolved otherwise. More especially, patients with severe depressive illness or other stressful state may present with 'Pseudo-Cushing's syndrome', but the insulin tolerance test is normal and so distinguishes this condition from true Cushing's syndrome.

If one or more screening tests prove positive, the patient should be admitted to the ward for more detailed investigations. In view of the strong clinical indication for Cushing's syndrome in this patient, the excessive excretion of urinary cortisol is unlikely to be due to a single episode of stress and may, therefore, be taken as conclusive evidence, so making other screening tests superfluous.

One of the cardinal biochemical abnormalities of Cushing's syndrome is the loss of circadian rhythm of cortisol secretion, but it does not usually become apparent unless blood specimens are collected over 24 hours and particularly at night, when cortisol secretion is normally at its lowest level. It must be borne in mind that the rhythm may be temporarily disturbed by the stress of admission to the ward or other illnesses. Hence plasma cortisol should be determined, 48 hours after admission, at 09.00 and 24.00 hours: if the two values fall in the same range, Cushing's syndrome is indicated. A valuable alternative, especially in children, is the determination of cortisol in small samples of mixed saliva. While the relationship between total plasma and the salivary hormone is non-linear, the cortisol content of saliva accurately reflects the level of free steroid in the plasma.

Differential diagnosis

With overproduction of cortisol confirmed, it is necessary to establish the cause, which could be either an excessive secretion of ACTH or autonomous hyperactivity of the adrenal cortex. A pituitary tumour, itself the result of excessive suprapituitary stimulation in the majority of cases, could be the source of the ACTH: this is Cushing's disease, which accounts for 70–80 per cent of cases of Cushing's syndrome. The presence of a space-occupying pituitary tumour sometimes manifests itself in enlargement of the pituitary fossa and encroachment of the sella turcica, not observed in the patient under discussion.

ACTH, or larger peptides containing the ACTH sequence, can be produced by a variety of extra-pituitary tumours located mostly in the thoracic cavity. The ACTH or parent peptide acts on the adrenal cortex in the usual manner but its secretion is not subject to feedback inhibition. The condition constitutes the ectopic ACTH syndrome and may present clinically in a form indistinguishable from the other variants of Cushing's syndrome. Sometimes the most prominent feature is a hypokalaemic alkalosis (*see* p. 37).

Overproduction of immunoreactive ACTH of whatever source

can be easily established by measuring the plasma hormone by radioimmunoassay. This assay usually yields higher values than the technically complex bioassay, probably owing to the presence of biologically inactive but immunoreactive fragments. Since a normally functioning pituitary would cease to secrete ACTH in the face of hypercortisolaemia, absence of plasma ACTH indicates unequivocally an adrenal origin of Cushing's syndrome. On the other hand, the presence of ACTH establishes Cushing's disease or the ectopic ACTH syndrome, higher plasma levels favouring the latter. However, immunoreactivity and biological activity are not synonymous and the presence in the plasma of biologically inactive but immunoreactive fragments produced by a tumour may have little or no clinical relevance.

While the direct ACTH assay is the test of choice, it is not always available. In that case, metyrapone can be used to differentiate Cushing's disease from other aetiologies of Cushing's syndrome. The drug, when given in large doses over 24 hours, blocks adrenal 11-hydroxylase and hence cortisol synthesis, but the possibility of severe side effects should limit the use of this test to cases in which diagnosis is not possible otherwise. Feedback inhibition of the hypothalamic-pituitary system will be largely lifted and hence ACTH secretion increased. The effect of this increased ACTH output from the pituitary will be to stimulate a normal adrenal to produce more cortisol precursors, e.g., 11-deoxycortisol or other 17-oxogenic steroids (17-OGS). The largely autonomous neoplastic adrenal will show little or no response, the non-tumorous parts of the cortex having atrophied as a result of prolonged suppression of ACTH, while the adrenal chronically exposed to ectopic ACTH cannot increase its output any more. Only the adrenal of Cushing's disease retains sufficient synthetic capacity to increase its pre-drug output substantially under additional ACTH stimulation (*Figure 5.1*).

Of the 20–30 per cent of patients with Cushing's syndrome of adrenal origin one half have adenomas, the other half carcinomas. A test based on partial suppression of urinary cortisol precursor output after 6-hourly administration of 2 mg dexamethasone for 2 days (high-dose dexamethasone test) often separates these patients from those with Cushing's disease (98 per cent) who usually manifest a substantial fall. The test is flawed, however, as it may be falsely positive or negative owing to spontaneous cyclic changes in cortisol production. Demonstration of reproducibility is therefore necessary. An abdominal X-ray may show calcification, usually of an adrenal carcinoma, and a CAT scan may indicate on which side the tumour

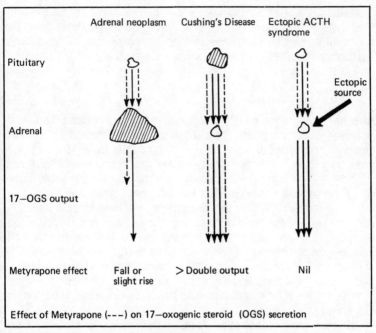

Pituitary

Adrenal

17—OGS output

Metyrapone effect   Fall or   >Double output   Nil
                   slight rise

Effect of Metyrapone (---) on 17—oxogenic steroid (OGS) secretion

Figure 5.1 Differential diagnosis of Cushing's Syndrome

is located, and possibly an ectopic source of ACTH. Downward displacement of one kidney, seen on an IV pyelogram, will also show which adrenal is affected. In contrast, overstimulation by ACTH, of whatever source, will result in bilateral adrenal hyperplasia.

It is axiomatic that any one test may be impossible to interpret because of atypical responses. Differentiation between pituitary and ectopic production can, on occasion, be particularly difficult. In the latter the disease takes a much more rapid clinical course and the overproduction of cortisol often does not manifest the usual stigmata owing to a loss of weight and early death of such patients. It is more likely to present with ACTH-induced hypokalaemia, manifesting as muscular weakness, and pigmentation, or with thirst and polyuria due to diabetes mellitus. Hypokalaemic alkalosis (K<3·3mmol. ℓ^{-1}, HCO$_3$>30 mmol. ℓ^{-1}, pH ≥7·50), due to excessive potassium loss and consequent intracellular acidosis, and diabetes are commonly associated with carcinoid tumours and are unusual in other types of Cushing's syndrome.

Radiological examination for tumours is always carried out in Cushing's syndrome together with CAT scanning, bronchoscopy and sputum cytology. An ovarian tumour suspected of producing cortisol may be detectable by pelvic examination.

Treatment

Adrenal tumours are mostly unilateral and the contralateral adrenal is likely to be atrophic. They frequently synthesize only modest amounts of cortisol and hence they are usually quite large by the time they have attracted attention by the stigmata of Cushing's syndrome. If a bilateral exploratory operation shows no visible signs of adenoma and provided that the preoperative diagnosis firmly points at the adrenals as the primary cause, both glands must be resected in the expectation that microadenomas will be found on histological examination. This conundrum underlines the crucial importance of the correct diagnosis prior to surgical intervention.

Glucocorticoid substitution therapy after the operation is essential and must be continued until the pituitary recovers from the prolonged feedback inhibition and the atrophic adrenal becomes functional once more.

Bilateral adrenalectomy entails indefinite treatment with glucocorticoids, salt and fludrocortisone. Non-resectable adrenal carcinomas sometimes respond to the cytotoxic drug o,p'-DDD, but eventually the tumour invades neighbouring organs and proceeds on its fatal course.

It is now known that *Cushing's disease* is usually caused by pituitary microadenomas. If they can be located and removed, a cure can be achieved without inducing deficiencies of other pituitary hormones. If the microadenoma cannot be found or is inaccessible (20–30 per cent of cases), total removal of the pituitary is a possibility. A preferred course is pituitary irradiation which does not cause deficiency of other hormones while destroying the adenoma, at least in juveniles (80 per cent), but only in 20 per cent of adults.

An alternative to pituitary surgery or irradiation is bilateral adrenalectomy which has often to be followed with radiation to the pituitary to prevent later development of neoplasm (Nelson's syndrome) otherwise occurring in 30 per cent of cases. The syndrome is marked by severe skin pigmentation as a consequence of the melanotropic effect of ACTH which rises to extremely high levels. The pituitary lesion is often malignant and the output of its hormone is autonomous. In the absence of irradiation it is therefore desirable to monitor the patient's plasma ACTH at intervals after adrenalectomy in order to detect any increase at the earliest moment. Selected cases of Cushing's disease have responded well to 'medical adrenalectomy' with o,p'-DDD, supported by dexamethasone to provide basic steroid cover.

A wide variety of tumours can be the source of *ectopic ACTH* but the single most common is oat cell carcinoma of the lung which is normally inoperable and insensitive to radiotherapy.

Additional Questions

1. Why is pigmentation a feature of both Cushing's syndrome and Addison's disease?
2. What are 17-oxogenic steroids (17-OGS)? Why is it more informative to measure urinary 17-OGS than 17-oxosteroids?

Further Reading

Liddle, G. W. (1981), Cushing's Syndrome, *Textbook of Endocrinology*, ed. Williams, R. H. 6th edn, pp. 267–276, W. B. Saunders Co., Philadelphia.

Case 6

Case History

Mrs. A. K., a 40-year-old civil servant, was admitted to hospital for investigation of persistent anaemia and complaints of 'bone tenderness'. She had had loose stools since she was 28 and she had suffered from fatigue, weight loss and abdominal cramps. Following each of two pregnancies at age 31 and 33 the diarrhoea had increased and she had noted swelling of the legs lasting several months. Her periods were irregular with 'average' losses. Three years prior to admission the patient experienced generalized bone pain, especially in the back, ribs and legs. Anaemia had been diagnosed by her GP who had treated her with oral iron for the past 6 months with no improvement. The patient had also suffered from depression for several years.

Examination

The patient was a thin, anxious lady, clinically anaemic. Height 158cm, weight 46 kg, Temperature 36·7 °C. Her tongue was red and sore and the corners of her mouth cracked. Several ecchymoses were scattered over her body.
CVS   Pulse 120 per minute, regular.
       Blood pressure 95/60 mm Hg (lying)
RS   Respiratory rate 22 per minute. Chest clear.
AS   Abdomen distended. Increased bowel sounds. No masses or tenderness.
LS   No lymphadenopathy.
All other systems: no abnormality detected.

Laboratory Investigations

Investigation	Result	Reference range
Haemoglobin (g/dl)	7·2	13·0 – 17·0
Serum K (mmol ℓ^{-1})	2·8	3·3 – 5·3
Serum iron (μmol ℓ^{-1})	7	13 – 32
Serum iron binding capacity (μmol ℓ^{-1})	80	45 – 70
Serum urea (mmol ℓ^{-1})	4·5	2·5 – 7·5
Serum total protein (g ℓ^{-1})	52	62 – 82

Continued on next page

Laboratory Investigations contd

Investigation	Result	Reference Range
Serum albumin (g ℓ^{-1})	25	35 – 50
Serum calcium (mmol ℓ^{-1})	1·75	2·25 – 2·65
Serum alkaline phosphatase (IU ℓ^{-1})	160	30 – 110
Serum phosphate (mmol ℓ^{-1})	0·6	0·8 – 1·6
Prothrombin time (sec.)	22	12 – 16

Questions

1. What is the differential diagnosis?
2. Are there any other investigations you would request?

Leading Questions

1. (a) Can the anaemia be defined in the light of the laboratory findings and the iron therapy?
   (b) Is this type of anaemia in accord with the other laboratory data?
   (c) Why is the alkaline phosphatase raised?
   (d) Can you suggest a cause for the bone pain?
   (e) Is there a single disease or syndrome which would link all these findings?
   (f) What are the possible aetiologies of the disease or syndrome?
   (g) Are any of the possible aetiologies less likely in view of the result of the clinical examination?
   (h) Could careful questioning of the patient eliminate some and make others more probable?
2. (a) What information can be obtained from examination of the faeces?
   (b) Are there any tests which would define the functional defect more precisely?
   (c) How would you investigate the reason for the bone pain?
   (d) Does the anaemia demand any further explanation?
   (e) What are the two possible reasons for the increased prothrombin time? How could you decide which is operative?
   (f) Hypoalbuminaemia is either due to inadequate synthesis or excessive loss; which is applicable in this patient?
   (g) Are there any other procedures which may be helpful in making a positive diagnosis?

Discussion

Here is a premenopausal woman presenting with weight loss, bone pain, anaemia which fails to respond to oral iron, and a long history of loose stools. The chronic nature of the latter does not suggest bacterial dysentery or cancer as a primary disease. Malabsorption is the most likely cause of her four cardinal signs and symptoms.

There are many causes of the malabsorption syndrome to be considered in this patient. They can be grouped into four broad classes:

1. Inadequate intraluminal digestion, e.g., pancreatic insufficiency and deficiency of bile salts due to liver and biliary tract disease or bile salt deconjugation as in blind loops, jejunal diverticula and fistulae.
2. Mucosal abnormalities (e.g., coeliac disease, Whipple's disease, Crohn's disease, amyloidosis).
3. Infection (e.g., tropical sprue, parasitosis).
4. Drugs (e.g., laxatives).

Generalized malabsorption

The biochemical abnormalities point to generalized malabsorption involving all types of substances. Thus, despite 6 months of oral therapy, the serum iron is low and the iron binding capacity is raised, which clearly indicates a failure of iron to be absorbed and probably accounts for the anaemia, although other factors such as B_{12} and folate deficiency and failure to absorb amino acids could contribute to it. Hypoalbuminaemia may well be another manifestation of inadequate amino acid supply to satisfy synthetic requirements, provided albuminuria and other losses of albumin can be ruled out. It explains the recurring ankle oedema. In so far as the hypocalcaemia does not merely reflect the low serum albumin, it, too, is likely to be due to failure of absorption, especially as there is no evidence of abnormal renal function. (The serum urea is within normal limits). Low serum calcium triggers parathyroid hormone secretion which would stimulate osteoclastic and osteoblastic activity, so accounting for the raised alkaline phosphatase.

The clinical findings fully support these tentative conclusions. Osteomalacia due to calcium and vitamin D deficiency is likely to be the cause of the bone pain, while glossitis, cheilosis and ecchymoses testify to malabsorption of B and C vitamins and of iron. Fermentation of unabsorbed food in the large gut can cause abnormal bowel sounds, gaseous distention and cramping abdominal pain.

Infection, defective digestion or absorption?

The absence of fever and abdominal tenderness or palpable mass lessen the likelihood of lymphatic obstruction, e.g., by small bowel lymphoma or TB. Careful questioning of the patient should provide information on her bowel habits in childhood, family history, previous illnesses and particularly surgical operations, which may suggest long-standing disorders, e.g., coeliac disease or complications following abdominal surgery. Dietary habits, including alcohol and drug abuse, must also be established. The choice of further laboratory tests is governed by the need to differentiate between defective digestion due to deficiency of pancreatic enzymes or of bile salts, defective absorption referable to disease of the intestinal wall, and malnutrition associated with bacterial and parasitic infections. In a patient with longstanding malabsorption and not recently returned from the tropics the last of these three broad classes is unlikely to be implicated.

Value of faecal examination

Examination of the stools is probably the most obvious requirement. Bulky, pale, fatty and malodorous stools suggest steatorrhoea which must be assessed by measuring the fat content of a 72 hour stool collection on a controlled fat intake. However, steatorrhoea is present in all major classes of the malabsorption syndrome, except for the primary mucosal abnormalities like lactase deficiency, and hence is non-discriminatory. Microscopic examination for parasites may usefully be done at this stage and a demonstration of occult blood would point to Crohn's disease or ulcerative colitis. If failure of fat absorption is coupled with defective absorption of mono-saccharide, which is independent of pancreatic enzymes, a mucosal defect is indicated. Thus an oral xylose absorption test showing a flat curve or reduced urinary excretion of xylose indicate such a defect.

Other investigations

A chest X-ray may give some indication of osteomalacia and enable pulmonary TB to be excluded, while X-rays of the upper GI tract and the small bowel, with and without barium, may show diverticula, fistulae and blind loops. Dilatation of the proximal jejunum with 'flocculation' of the barium points strongly at adult coeliac disease, although Whipple's disease and amyloidosis may present a similar picture. Chronic pancreatitis is unlikely in the absence of epigastric pain, pancreatic calcification or a history of alcohol abuse. We know that the patient's anaemia is partly due to failure to absorb iron, but determination of serum and red cell folate, serum B_{12} and possibly a bone marrow would indicate whether B_{12} and folate deficiencies contribute to the pathology, especially in view of the possible link between vitamin B complex deficiency and glossitis and cheilosis. Fat-soluble vitamins (K and D) also will be poorly absorbed, so accounting for the bleeding tendency and the osteomalacia. Hypocalcaemia is due to the negative calcium balance arising from loss of both endogenous and dietary calcium in the diarrhoeal fluid where it is sequestered by free fatty acids to form insoluble calcium soap, and from vitamin D deficiency and hence poor absorption.

The diarrhoeal losses of K^+ explain the low plasma level of the ion. Liver function tests may be necessary if malabsorption does not adequately account for the hypoprothrombinaemia or hypo-albuminaemia. It should be noted, however, that in most if not all intestinal mucosal diseases, with or without ulceration, plasma proteins are lost by leakage into the gut lumen, in addition to a reduced hepatic synthesis engendered by poor absorption of amino acids.

Intestinal biopsy

Finally, a peroral jejunal biopsy may give valuable aid in the differential diagnosis of the malabsorption syndrome and is easily and safely performed with a Crosby capsule, provided the pro-thrombin time is normal. Partial or complete villous atrophy is a characteristic feature of coeliac disease, but it is occasionally found also in tropical sprue and a variety of other intestinal diseases. Whipple's disease may be diagnosed by the demonstration of macrophages laden with glycoprotein in the lamina propria of the intestinal wall, while deposits of amyloid in the submucosa confirm amyloidosis. Parasites have occasionally been found in jejunal biopsies.

Treatment

Treatment of the malabsorption syndrome, and its success, obviously depends on the aetiology of the disorder. Coeliac disease usually responds dramatically to a gluten-free diet, with improvement in the histological appearance of the intestinal mucosa and normalisation of absorption. The toxicity of gluten resides in small peptides of 5000–10 000 daltons against which the immunological defences appear defective. However, even on a gluten-'free' diet (observance of which is difficult to verify) the bacterial flora of the small intestine may remain abnormal and consume nutrients normally available to the host, as well as interfering with digestion and absorption. The factors conducive to changes in the bacterial flora, common to all classes of the malabsorption syndrome, are the presence of unabsorbed food constituents, decreased mobility, mucosal lesions and defective local immunological defence.

Pancreatic insufficiency requires replacement of digestive enzymes and insulin in cases where the endocrine function of the organ is impaired, as well as treatment of the underlying cause. Some diseases of the liver and biliary tract leading to a deficiency of bile acid and hence defective fat absorption may be treated surgically (fistula or obstruction of bile flow), in others supportive treatment with fat-soluble vitamins and calcium counteracts the osteoporosis and osteomalacia which are a common sequela of bile salt deficiency. Strictures, diverticula and blind loops often harbour bacteria which deconjugate bile acids and so have a similar effect on fat absorption. They may be amenable to surgical correction or long-term antimicrobial treatment. The latter is effective also in Whipple's disease, if maintained indefinitely. Essentially empirical and supportive therapy is the only recourse in Crohn's disease and amyloidosis.

Chronic depression, fatigue and lack of drive are frequent features of the malabsorption syndrome and sometimes the main presenting symptoms. They often disappear without specific treatment if the underlying malabsorption is repaired.

Additional Questions

1. Which foods would you expect to exacerbate the diarrhoea in coeliac disease?
2. Which of the suggested further tests would be normal in pancreatic insufficiency?

Further Reading

Sleisenger, M. H. and Brandborg, L. L. (1977). *Malabsorption*, W. B. Saunders, Co., Philadelphia.

Case 7

Case History

M.W., a 76-year-old widow, who had previously been well was referred to the local chest clinic with a recent history of four episodes of haemoptysis. She had no other symptoms. At the clinic she was found to be severely hypertensive and was admitted to hospital urgently for investigation and treatment.

Examination

The patient was fit for her age and was not anaemic, cyanosed or jaundiced.
CVS   Pulse 80 per minute regular.
            Blood pressure 230/120 mm Hg (lying).
            Heart sounds: loud first sound.
RS   Few scattered rhonchi otherwise clear.
All other systems: no abnormality detected.
Chest X-ray   Lung fields clear, no evidence of malignancy.
ECG   Left axis deviation.

Laboratory investigations

Investigation	Result	Reference range
Plasma sodium (mmol. ℓ^{-1})	143	135 – 145
Plasma potassium (mmol. ℓ^{-1})	2·7	3·5 – 5·5
Plasma chloride (mmol. ℓ^{-1})	96	98 – 108
Plasma HCO_3 (mmol. ℓ^{-1})	33	22 – 30
Plasma urea (mmol. ℓ^{-1})	3·0	2·5 – 7·5
Serum bilirubin (μmol. ℓ^{-1})	12	<20
Serum alkaline phosphatase (IU. ℓ^{-1})	35	30 – 110
Serum alanine aminotransferase (IU. ℓ^{-1})	37	15 – 55
Serum total protein (g. ℓ^{-1})	71	62 – 82
Serum albumin (g. ℓ^{-1})	36	35 – 50
Serum calcium (mmol. ℓ^{-1})	2·5	2·25 – 2·65
Serum phosphate (mmol. ℓ^{-1})	1·12	0·8 – 1·6
Urine sodium (mmol. 24 h^{-1})	58	110 – 240
Urine potassium (mmol. 24 h^{-1})	72	35 – 110

Questions

1. What is the relationship, if any, between the clinical and biochemical abnormalities?
2. What further investigations are required to establish the aetiology?

Leading Questions

1. (a) What is the presenting symptom?
   (b) Can this be related to any of the clinical findings in the patient?
   (c) Do the radiological findings help in narrowing the diagnostic possibilities?
   (d) Assuming adequate dietary intake of potassium, loss of this ion from the ECF is the only alternative explanation for the hypokalaemia. What are the three major routes by which potassium may leave the extracellular space?
   (e) Can any of these be ruled out (i) on clinical grounds, (ii) on the basis of potassium excretion in the urine or (iii) in the light of other biochemical data?
   (f) Having excluded a number of possible causes of hypokalaemia (with inappropriate potassium excretion), can the most likely cause be linked with the patient's hypertension?
2. (a) Which hormones are involved in normal potassium regulation?
   (b) In what pathological conditions can other hormones interfere with this regulation?
   (c) Are there any drugs or other substances which can mimic any of these hormones?

Discussion

The two striking findings in this patient who presents with a history of haemoptysis are the high blood pressure found on clinical examination and the low plasma potassium in the laboratory investigation. Haemoptysis is a rare complication of hypertension but the negative findings in the other laboratory tests and in the clinical and radiological examinations increases the probability that the hypertension could in fact be the cause. In many cases presenting with haemoptysis the aetiology is not immediately found and other causes can not finally be ruled out until the patient has been followed up for several months.

Physiology of potassium

It is therefore necessary to investigate the hypokalaemia and its relationship to the hypertension to arrive at a diagnosis. The differential diagnosis of hypokalaemia demands a brief review of normal potassium physiology. Potassium is distributed in the body in such a manner that 98 per cent of the ion is in the intracellular (IC) space, particularly in muscle, at a concentration of 125 mmol. kg^{-1}. The remaining 2 per cent is in the extracellular fluid (ECF) and plasma. Plasma potassium concentration can reflect changes in intake and output and also shifts of the ion between the IC and EC compartments. More than one factor may be operating in a patient simultaneously and affect the plasma potassium concentration in opposite directions. A shift of a small fraction of IC potassium to the EC compartment will cause a substantial rise in plasma potassium. On the other hand a much larger proportion of the EC potassium must move into cells to produce hypokalaemia giving rise to only a small relative increase in the IC concentration. The result of either of these shifts is to cause a substantial change in the IC:EC potassium ratio which leads to alteration in the cell membrane electrical potential and in turn to many of the symptoms of hypokalaemia and hyperkalaemia.

In view of the relative distribution and transfer of the ion between the IC and EC fluids, the plasma potassium concentration is not always a reliable indicator of total body potassium and in various pathological conditions IC potassium can be severely depleted while the plasma potassium remains normal. These include diabetic ketoacidosis, chronic congestive cardiac failure, cirrhosis and uraemia. On the other hand hypokalaemia can exist in some conditions in which total body potassium is normal, e.g., familial periodic paralysis in which there is a temporary shift of potassium into cells. The plasma potassium concentration must, therefore, be interpreted in conjunction with all the known facts on the clinical and metabolic state of the patient.

Causes of hypokalaemia

Decreased intake of potassium (which is widely distributed in foods), rarely causes hypokalaemia but it can exacerbate potassium losing conditions. The major cause of hypokalaemia is loss of potassium either from the gastrointestinal or renal tracts. Substantial potassium losses can occur in the sweat. Intestinal secretions contain large quantities of potassium and losses occur through vomiting, drainage of biliary, intestinal or pancreatic fistulae and diarrhoea. Severe intestinal potassium losses can occur through excessive use of laxatives or enemas. A rare cause of hypokalaemia is found in patients with ureterosigmoidostomies in which the bowel wall secretes potassium in exchange for sodium. Alternatively, plasma can be lost from the ECF by transfer to the ICF.

The patient gave no history of intestinal symptoms and denied taking laxatives. A gastro-intestinal cause for her hypokalaemia is therefore unlikely. The most probable aetiology is renal loss and this is confirmed by the presence of a considerable quantity of potassium in the urine which is unphysiological in the face of hypokalaemia. Filtered potassium is 80–90 per cent reabsorbed in the proximal tubule and the loop of Henlé. Potassium balance is maintained in the distal tubule and collecting duct in which the ion can be reabsorbed or secreted. Excretion of potassium is controlled by a number of factors including sodium balance, mineralocorticoid activity, changes in hydrogen ion concentration and urine flow. Diseases or other agents which alter these factors will cause potassium retention or loss and this can result in hyperkalaemia or hypokalaemia respectively.

Patients with renal failure usually have hyperkalaemia but potassium wasting can occur in a number of renal diseases including hereditary or acquired renal tubular acidosis (proximal or distal), pyelonephritis and in the diuretic phase of acute tubular necrosis. The patient under consideration shows no evidence of renal failure (normal plasma urea) or acidosis (high plasma bicarbonate) and hence these investigations together with the history and examination exclude a primary renal cause of hypokalaemia.

Role of mineralocorticoids

An increase in mineralocorticoid activity giving rise to sodium retention and potassium loss by the kidney can occur in a variety of conditions many of which are associated with hypertension. Primary hyperaldosteronism is most frequently a result of an adrenal adenoma or carcinoma. Secondary hyperaldosteronism is caused by a number of different conditions which stimulate the renin-angiotensin-aldosterone pathway. Patients in whom the prime stimulus is effective intravascular volume depletion, e.g., those with congestive cardiac failure, cirrhosis and nephrotic syndrome, are unlikely to develop hypertension. In other patients in whom the stimulus is reduction in renal blood flow, e.g., renal artery stenosis or malignant hypertension, increased activity of the renin-angiotensin-aldosterone pathway can cause or exacerbate hypertension. Hypokalaemia and hypertension are sometimes found in patients with Cushing's syndrome and in the 11-hydroxylase deficiency type of congenital adrenal hyperplasia. Differentiation of these conditions is based on clinical examination, radiology and measurements of plasma electrolytes, GFR and where necessary urine free cortisol, plasma renin and aldosterone. The presence of hypertension almost certainly excludes volume depletion and the renal tubular problems in the patient. However several of the other causes of increased mineralocorticoid activity cannot be excluded and further investigation would have had to be pursued had not the diagnosis come to light.

A number of drugs can cause hypokalaemia by increasing renal losses. In the main they are the thiazide and loop diuretics which produce their effect by inhibiting sodium reabsorption. The increased sodium load presented to the distal nephron promotes sodium-potassium exchange which can lead to hypokalaemia. However in practice only 7 per cent of patients treated with diuretics have a plasma potassium $<3{\cdot}0$ mmol. ℓ^{-1}. Routine potassium supplements are, therefore, not required and the value of repeated electrolyte determinations in patients on diuretics is questionable. A second group of drugs are those with mineralocorticoid activity, including carbenoxolone used in the treatment of gastric ulcer. This drug is related to glycyrrhizic acid which is found in liquorice root and which when taken in large amounts also gives rise to hypokalaemia and hypertension. An astute SHO elicited a history of liquorice addiction from the patient after the discovery of the low plasma potassium, thus saving her from extensive investigation.

Sequelae of hypokalaemia

The metabolic consequences of potassium depletion are wide-spread but variable and can involve kidney, myocardium, nervous system and gastrointestinal tract. The patient showed none of the expected ECG abnormalities: depressed ST segment, inversion of T waves and accentuated U waves. She did have a metabolic alkalosis (raised pH and plasma bicarbonate) which can both cause and be the result of hypokalaemia. In hypokalaemia there is a reduction in IC potassium which is lost from the cell down a concentration gradient. This has a twofold effect: in the distal tubule it results in an increased ability to reabsorb bicarbonate and, at the same time, it is probable that hydrogen ions move into cells. The increased hydrogen ion in the renal distal tubular cell is secreted into the urine. Both effects lead to an alkalosis. On the other hand reasons for hypokalaemia occuring as the result of a metabolic alkalosis are complex and depend in part on the cause and duration of the alkalosis. Increased sodium delivery to the distal tubule, the increase in pH itself and a selective increase in delivery of bicarbonate to the distal tubule all increase potassium excretion. Other postulated causes are osmotic diuresis and the activity of hormones.

Therapy in this case is simple, being withdrawal of the offending liquorice. Treatment can also be carried out with mineralocorticoid antagonists such as spironolactone and triamterene which cause potassium retention. Potassium is not required in this patient whose symptoms are mild but will be needed in more severely affected patients. If intravenous therapy is necessary great care must be taken and rates exceeding 40 mmol. h^{-1}, and high infusion concentrations must be avoided. ECG monitoring is advisable.

The patient made a rapid recovery on treatment, the plasma potassium concentration rose to 3·7 mmol. ℓ^{-1} within 5 days and the blood pressure fell to 150/90 mm Hg (lying) a few days later.

Additional Questions

1. In which of the following conditions is hypokalaemia associated with hypertension: laxative abuse, periodic paralysis, ectopic ACTH secreting tumour, diuretic therapy and Cushing's syndrome?
2. How does the plasma pH or bicarbonate help in the differential diagnosis?

Further Reading

Gennari, F. J. and Cohen, J. J. (1975) Role of the kidney in potassium homeostasis: lessons from acid-base disturbances (Editorial), *Kidney International*, **8**, pp. 1–5.

Lindeman, R. D., (1976) Hypokalaemia: causes, consequences and correction, *Am. J. Med. Sci.*, **272**, pp. 5–17.

Case 8

Case History

A. B., a male infant of Pakistani parents was born following a normal full term pregnancy and delivery. His mother (para 2 + 1) and father were first cousins. His birth weight was 4600 g. and the Apgar score was 9 at 1 and 5 minutes after birth. The baby was bottle fed. Progress was normal for the first 36 hours of life, the baby was then noted to have twitching limbs, staring eyes, cyanosis and a rapid respiratory rate. A blood glucose was measured on the ward from a heel prick sample using a glucose specific stick method. The result was 1·0 mmol. ℓ^{-1} and the baby was transferred to SCBU.

There was no relevant family history, both siblings were alive and well at 3 and 4 years of age respectively. Mother had had one early miscarriage at six weeks of pregnancy.

Examination (on SCBU)

The baby was large with both weight (4500 g.) and length (55 cm) above the 90th centile. Head circumference was 34 cm on the 50th centile. There was no fitting or cyanosis at the time of the examination. No obvious congenital abnormalities were noted. Temperature 38 °C.

CVS   Pulse 140 per minute regular.
        Heart sounds normal.
RS   Respiratory rate 90 per minute.
        Chest clear.
        No clinical evidence of pneumothorax.
No other findings of note.

Laboratory investigations

Initial tests

Investigation	Result	Reference range[a]
Plasma glucose (mmol. ℓ^{-1})	1·1	1·6 – 4·5
Plasma sodium (mmol. ℓ^{-1})	137	135 – 145
Plasma potassium (mmol. ℓ^{-1})	6·2	4·0 – 6·5
Plasma chloride (mmol. ℓ^{-1})	105	95 – 105

Continued on next page

Laboratory Investigations contd

Investigation	Result	Reference range
Plasma bicarbonate (mmol. ℓ^{-1})	19	18 – 27
Plasma urea (mmol. ℓ^{-1})	5·6	2·5 – 7·5
Plasma creatinine (μmol. ℓ^{-1})	110	57 – 100
Serum calcium (mmol. ℓ^{-1})	1·87	1·8 – 3·0
Serum magnesium (mmol. ℓ^{-1})	0·65	0·75 – 1·15
Serum phosphate (mmol. ℓ^{-1})	2·3	1·3 – 2·5
Serum bilirubin (μmol. ℓ^{-1})	53	70 – 110
Blood gases (capillary):		
pH	7·49	7·32 – 7·49
P_{CO_2} (mm Hg)	35	27 – 41
P_{O_2} (mm Hg)	76	60 – 80
Base excess (mmol. ℓ^{-1})	−2	−6 – 1
CSF glucose (mmol. ℓ^{-1})	0·8	40 – 80% concurrent plasma glucose
Haemoglobin (g. dl⁻¹)	17·7	15 – 24
White cell count ($\times 10^9$. ℓ^{-1})	10·7 (75% neutrophils)	7·25
Blood and CSF culture negative		

[a] Reference ranges are for a full term infant of appropriate age.

Further tests Urine and plasma amino acids, urine organic acids and screening test for galactosaemia all negative.
Plasma lactate 1·8 mmol. ℓ^{-1} (normal <3·0 mmol. ℓ^{-1}) Plasma ammonia 97 μmol. ℓ^{-1} (normal <80 μmol. ℓ^{-1})

Progress

The patient was treated with 10 – 15 per cent glucose IV, phenobarbitone and antibiotics. Despite this he suffered further severe hypoglycaemic episodes and continued to have frequent convulsions.

Questions

1. What is the differential diagnosis at the time of transfer to SCBU?
2. What are the possible causes of the major biochemical abnormality and how would further investigations help with the diagnosis?

Leading Questions

1. (a) What is the clinical problem which leads to the initial blood glucose measurement?
   (b) What are the four major causes of convulsions in the neonate? Can inferences be drawn from the age of first occurrence of a convulsion?
   (c) What relevant information can be obtained from the antenatal and birth histories?
   (d) Does the relationship between the parents favour one group of diagnoses?
   (e) On what regulatory mechanisms and other factors does maintenance of normoglycaemia depend?
2. (a) What metabolic defects can cause neonatal hypoglycaemia?
   (b) Can any of these defects be excluded on the basis of the initial laboratory tests?
   (c) What further investigations can help to confirm or exclude other metabolic defects?
   (d) What endocrine abnormalities could account for the hypoglycaemia observed in the patient?
   (e) Are there circumstances in which such abnormalities could be transient?
   (f) What additional investigations are needed to establish an endocrine cause of the hypoglycaemia?

Discussion

Convulsion in the neonatal period is a paediatric emergency which can have many different causes among which brain damage due to perinatal trauma or hypoxia, metabolic disorders, infection and developmental abnormalities account for the great majority. With changes in obstetric and neonatal practice, the contribution of birth trauma and hypoxia has been reduced and that of metabolic derangements has proportionately increased. The most common cause of neonatal convulsions varies with the gestational and post-natal age of the child. Perinatal complications following birth trauma and hypoxia and intracranial haemorrhage account for the majority of early convulsions particularly in premature infants. In the full term, normal weight infant metabolic causes present most frequently between the fourth and eighth days when a deficiency or excess of a metabolite develops. If the baby is of low birth weight or premature, deficiencies of metabolites are likely to develop earlier, while delays in feeding can postpone the accumulation of toxic metabolites. Convulsions associated with septicaemia tend to occur in the second half of the first week of life. In some cases the history, including antenatal history, together with a clinical examination will reveal the diagnosis but most convulsing neonates will require investigation, including biochemical, haematological and micro-biological tests as well as radiology.

Problems with the interpretation of tests

The interpretation of routine biochemical tests in these patients is difficult, not least because glucose, calcium, magnesium, phosphate or sodium may be found to be abnormal in 90 per cent of neonates with convulsions of different aetiologies. Hypoglycaemia or hypocalcaemia may be a primary cause of the convulsions or may be secondary to a disorder associated with fits; they may be due to cerebral anoxia or oedema and intracranial haemorrhage, while hypoglycaemia may occur in patients with developmental abnormalities. Other factors in interpreting the biochemical findings are gestational and postnatal age and birth weight which can affect the reference ranges with which the actual values should be compared. For example a blood glucose of $<1\cdot1$ mol. ℓ^{-1} (<20 mg/dl) is considered diagnostically significant in premature babies while the equivalent value for full term infants is $<1\cdot6$ mmol. ℓ^{-1} (<30 mg/dl). Likewise the normal mean calcium concentration in premature infants in the first week of life is 0·25 mmol. ℓ^{-1} (1 mg/dl) lower than in full term babies. Calcium concentrations are also related to diet; babies fed on cows milk preparations have lower serum calcium concentrations than breast fed babies. This is due to the high phosphate content of cows milk which raises the serum phosphate and secondarily depresses the calcium and is particularly prevalent at the end of the first week of life when hypocalcaemic convulsions predominate.

The slightly raised plasma creatinine and ammonia and lowered magnesium in this baby are not of great significance. The major finding was the severe hypoglycaemia which proved resistant to treatment with glucose. Maintenance of normoglycaemia in the neonate is complex, depending on endocrinological, metabolic and environmental factors. At birth the infant liver has a very high glycogen content and the blood glucose concentration reflects the maternal value. Postnatally there is a rapid fall in blood glucose as homeostatic mechanisms come into play and the body relies on breakdown of liver glycogen stimulated by glucagon and catecholamines. In fact, the blood glucose concentration is somewhat labile in the following 48 hours depending on factors such as feeding (especially the first feed), ambient temperature and handling of the baby (e.g., in the taking of repeated blood specimens to assess hypoglycaemia!). Normal babies also have substantial reserves of fat and during the first week of life the enzymes of fatty acid catabolism become active and fat becomes the main energy source; this is reflected in a drop in the respiratory quotient from 1·0 to 0·7. If fat is absent, as in premature babies or those of low birth weight, then this will increase demand on the limited carbohydrate stores and predispose the infant to hypoglycaemia.

The choice of sample and method for measurement of blood glucose is important. The rate of glycolysis of neonatal red cells is greater compared with older children and adults; hence it is important that blood be analyzed immediately or, if stored even for a short time, an inhibitor of glycolysis is essential. Glucose concentrations in whole blood are approximately 15 per cent less than in plasma. Also, there is marked individual variation in the blood/plasma glucose ratios and hence plasma is preferred for analysis. If the peripheral circulation is good there is a negligible difference in glucose measured in venous or capillary specimens. However, many convulsing neonates will have poor capillary blood flow and in this case a spuriously low glucose concentration may be found. Finally, it should be emphasised that although normally the correlation between ward testing using dip stick and laboratory glucose measurements is quite good, it is poor at low concentrations and the stick methods should never be relied on either for diagnosis or management.

Possible causes of hypoglycaemia

As well as the circumstances mentioned above in which the hypo-glycaemia is secondary to other conditions causing convulsions, a number of specific disorders give rise to neonatal hypoglycaemia and convulsions. The hypoglycaemia results from increased utiliza-tion and/or decreased production of glucose. Transient neonatal hypoglycaemia occurs most frequently in babies who are small for gestational age and also in infants of diabetic mothers or with erythroblastosis. Antenatal complications, particularly toxaemia and high blood pressure, are found in half of these cases and boys are three times more often affected than girls. The antenatal, birth and postnatal history, the clinical examination and the persistent nature of the hypoglycaemia in this infant make the diagnosis of transient neonatal hypoglycaemia unlikely.

When hypoglycaemia is severe, persistent and unresponsive to glucose therapy, a metabolic or endocrine cause is likely. Obviously deficiencies of the enzymes of glycogenolysis or gluconeogenesis can lead to hypoglycaemia e.g. deficiencies of phosphorylase, glucose-6-phosphatase, fructose-1-6-diphospha-tase and pyruvate dehydrogenase. However, many other inborn errors of carbohydrate and amino acid metabolism can present with hypoglycaemia as one of the initial biochemical findings. It is essen-tial in these cases to measure plasma and urine amino acids, urine organic acids, plasma ammonia and lactate and blood gases to screen for these potential causes of hypoglycaemia. All these tests were negative in this patient and an endocrine cause for his hypo-glycaemia is therefore the probable diagnosis.

Hormonal regulation

The endocrine control of glucose homeostasis is by the opposing actions of insulin which lowers blood glucose on the one hand and cortisol (and ACTH), growth hormone and glucagon which raise it. Glucocorticoid insufficiency in congenital adrenal hyperplasia is probably the commonest endocrine abnormality. The hypogly-caemia in infants of diabetic mothers and those with erythroblastosis is due to transient hyperinsulinism which results more permanently from pancreatic islet B cell abnormalities. Whatever the cause of hyperinsulinism, these babies are often large which can be a useful clinical clue. The diagnosis depends on the measurement of insulin and/or C-peptide during a hypoglycaemic episode. In normal infants as the blood glucose concentration falls there is a parallel fall in insulin and C-peptide but in hyperinsulinism hormone secretion is inappropriately high for the glucose concentration, even when the actual insulin values fall within the normal fasting reference range. It cannot be emphasised too strongly that the hormone values must be interpreted with respect to the simultaneous blood glucose measurement. (Similar considerations must be borne in mind with other hormones, e.g., parathyroid hormone and ACTH, whose concentrations must be interpreted in relation to calcium and cortisol respectively.)

The insulin and C-peptide were measured urgently in this patient and the results below confirmed hyperinsulinism:

Age	2 days	3 days	Reference range (fasting)
Insulin (mU. ℓ^{-1})	19	15	<10
C-peptide (pmol. ℓ^{-1})	1·8	1·6	<0·6
Glucose (mmol. ℓ^{-1})	1·1	1·0	1·6 – 4·5

An inference of hyperinsulinism as the cause of hypoglycaemia can be made, even if insulin or C-peptide cannot be assayed, on the basis of the following indicators:

1. Hypoglycaemic episodes are not accompanied by ketosis
2. Normoglycaemia cannot be achieved except by high and continuous rates of glucose infusion
3. The patient's hypoglycaemia responds to glucagon.

The histological findings in these patients vary from single B cell tumours through multiple islet abnormalities to functional B cell disorders, all of which are referred to by the general term of nesidioblastosis. There is an effective increase in B cell activity and interestingly a reduction in somatostatin-secreting cells which may predispose to increased insulin secretion. Clinical presentation is similar in all varieties of nesidioblastosis.

Treatment of mild cases of nesidioblastosis is with frequent and regular feeding by day and night. In severe cases diazoxide is used with a thiazide diuretic. Diazoxide depresses insulin secretion and the thiazide diuretic raises the blood sugar by an extra-pancreatic mechanism. If medical treatment fails, subtotal and even complete pancreatectomy may be needed, following which the patient will need replacement of insulin and pancreatic enzymes.

Additional Questions

1. What is the role of somatostatin?
2. Why is ketosis absent in hypoglycaemia associated with hyper-insulinism?

Further Reading

Marks, V. and Rose, F. C. (1981) *Hypoglycaemia*, 2nd Edn, pp. 266–323, Blackwell Scientific Publications, Oxford.
Volpe, J. (1973), Neonatal Seizures, *N. Engl. J. Med.*, **289**, pp. 413–416.

Case 9

Case History

Jennifer J., a 23-year-old medical student, was admitted to hospital 10 days after returning from an elective period in West Africa. She complained of anorexia, nausea, vomiting, headache, weakness and a persistent dull abdominal pain in the right upper quadrant. Her temperature fluctuated between 37·5 °C and 38.5 °C and in the last 2 days her urine had become dark. Following admission the symptoms gradually subsided over a period of 3 weeks.

Examination

On admission the patient was mildly jaundiced but not anaemic.
Temperature 38·2 °C.
CVS   Pulse 84 regular; BP 120/80 mm Hg (lying).
AS   Liver enlarged 3 cm, tender.
LS   Cervical lymph nodes enlarged.
All other systems: no abnormality detected.

Laboratory investigations

Investigation	Result Day 2	Day 7	Day 14	Day 21	Reference range
Haemoglobin (g/dl)	11·6	11·6	11·5	11·4	11·8 – 15·2
Red cells (10^{12}. ℓ^{-1})	4·0	4·0	3·8	3·8	3·9 – 5·3
White cells (10^9. ℓ^{-1})	8^a	8^a	8^a	8^a	4 – 11
Prothrombin time (sec)	17		$25(19)^b$	18	12 – 16
Alanine Aminotransferase (ALT) (IU. ℓ^{-1})	950	1500	980	475	15 – 55
Serum alkaline phosphatase (IU. ℓ^{-1})	190	550	720	420	30 – 110
Serum albumin (g. ℓ^{-1})	35		34	33	35 – 50
Serum bilirubin (μmol. ℓ^{-1})	40 (mainly conjugated)	85 (conjugated + unconjugated)	110 (conjugated + unconjugated)	70 (mainly unconjugated)	3 – 20
Urine bilirubin	+	+ +	+	0	0
Urine urobilinogen	+ +	+	0	0	(+)
Stools (colour)	normal	pale		normal	

^{a} Relative lymphocytosis; 5 per cent of lymphocytes are atypical
^{b} 24 hours after 10mg menadione subcutaneously.

Questions

1. What is the differential diagnosis?
2. What further tests should be/have been done?

Leading Questions

1. (a) What are the two most likely diagnostic possibilities in a young woman presenting with 'flu-like symptoms and jaundice?
   (b) Does the patient's stay in West Africa suggest another possible diagnosis?
   (c) Does the moderate lymphocytosis and the presence of atypical lymphocytes support one or other of the choices?
   (d) What factors determine prothrombin synthesis and hence the prothrombin time?
   (e) Do the haematological and biochemical data obtained on day 2 offer evidence for or against one particular type of jaundice?
   (f) Why is the urine dark?
   (g) Does the presence of the bilirubin in the urine corroborate one particular finding in the serum?
   (h) Where does urobilinogen originate? Does its presence at ++ level in the urine, together with the normal stool colour, offer evidence against one type of jaundice?
   (i) Are there any forms of hyperbilirubinaemia, not associated with disease, which should be considered?
   (j) What external agents, other than viruses, which cause jaundice ought to be especially considered in this patient?
   (k) In what circumstances does intracellular ALT leak out into the plasma? Would you expect parenchymal disease to be more or less prone than biliary obstruction to lead to such leakage?
   (l) Why is a high serum phosphatase indicative of cholestasis?
   (m) Why is the serum albumin low?
   (n) What conclusions can be drawn from the qualitative and quantitative changes in the serum and urine bilirubin manifested on days 7 and 14?
   (o) Why does the urobilinogen disappear from the urine in the course of the illness? How does this fit in with the pale stools?
   (p) Does the change in prothrombin time and the effect of menadione accord with other parameters?

(q) How would you interpret the biochemical changes from day 14 to 21?

(r) In the light of available clinical and laboratory data, what is the diagnosis?

2. (a) Which tests would have been appropriate in view of
    (i) the viral origin of the illness
    (ii) the stay in West Africa?

(b) In what circumstances is a needle biopsy of the liver definitely contraindicated?

(c) Would a plain X-ray have been helpful?

(d) Are there any other tests which could usefully be done after day 21?

Discussion

The presenting symptoms of headache, fever and lymph node enlargement in a young adult suggest infectious mononucleosis which is occasionally associated with hepatitis, as indicated by jaundice and a tender, enlarged liver. However, the absence of pharyngotonsillitis, which accompanies mononucleosis, may be more consistent with infectious hepatitis whose 'flu-like early symptoms often precede more definite signs of liver involvement. The pain in the right upper quadrant probably originates in the liver. Aversion to food, nausea and vomiting are referable to liver involvement but cast no light on the aetiology. On the other hand, the patient has just returned from an area where malaria is endemic and her symptoms are entirely compatible with this disease. Despite the nature of the pain, the possibility of extrahepatic or intrahepatic obstruction of bile flow must also be considered.

Haematological data obtained on day 2: the patient is clearly anaemic, a circumstance which might suggest haemolytic jaundice. A normal white cell count, with reduced granulocytes and relative lymphocytosis and some atypical lymphocytes, are consistent either with infectious mononucleosis or uncomplicated viral hepatitis. The slightly increased prothrombin time is due to defective synthesis of prothrombin or other hepatic clotting factors for reasons as yet unclear.

The biochemical data on day 2 confirm a mild hyperbilirubinaemia involving mainly conjugated bilirubin. This suggests a lesion distal to conjugation with glucuronic acid and effectively rules out haemolysis as a cause of the jaundice; its origin has to be further investigated. The dark colour of the urine must be due to conjugated bilirubin since the unconjugated pigment is insoluble in water and so cannot be excreted by the kidney. Urobilinogen, unlike its oxidation product urobilin (stercobilin), is colourless and hence its presence at + + level in the urine does not contribute to the dark colour. It is formed in the gut by bacterial reduction of bilirubin, and some of it is reabsorbed into the enterohepatic circulation and normally re-excreted by the liver to be finally oxidised in the gut to stercobilin which gives the faeces the brown colour. Since haemolytic jaundice is ruled out, the increased excretion of urobilinogen in the urine must be due to a specific failure of the liver to re-excrete the substance, thus implicating parenchymal liver damage rather than biliary obstruction as a cause of the hyperbilirubinaemia. The normal colour of the faeces offers support for this conclusion.

Other causes of jaundice must be considered. Gilbert's syndrome, due to defective uptake of bilirubin into the liver cells, manifests as unconjugated bilirubin in the serum. An impaired secretion of conjugated bilirubin and certain organic anions into the bile, the Dubin-Johnson syndrome, is characterized by elevation of both conjugated and unconjugated bilirubin in the serum. It is a harmless condition, although it may be associated with abdominal pain. Rotor's syndrome presents similarly and, like the other two, is familial and requires no treatment. None of these three inherited disorders are marked by any other biochemical abnormalities. Many drugs, including oral contraceptives, impair bilirubin transport and so lead to jaundice and careful questioning is necessary to eliminate this potential cause.

The activities of certain enzymes in the serum provide valuable additional clues to the nature, extent and persistence of liver disease. Alanine aminotransferase (ALT) is a particularly sensitive index of liver damage. The enzyme, although not specific for liver, is at least 10 times more abundant in that organ than in any other. It is present in the cytoplasm of the hepatocyte and if the cell membrane becomes abnormally permeable, the enzyme escapes, raising the serum level 20 or more times the upper limit of the reference range. Since ALT is not excreted in the bile to any considerable extent, a rise of that order in the serum level indicates hepatocellular damage. In inflammatory conditions such as hepatitis leakage of ALT is more pronounced than escape of a related enzyme, aspartate aminotransferase (AST) which is a mitochondrial as well as a cytoplasmic enzyme. On the other hand, in chronic liver damage or in gross cellular necrosis, e.g., in paracetamol poisoning, the serum AST rises to higher levels than the ALT.

On day 2 the serum ALT is 17 times the upper normal limit and it reaches a peak about one week after the onset of jaundice, declining fairly rapidly thereafter, in parallel with the clinical improvement. This picture is typical of hepatitis, recovery from which is not deemed to be complete until the ALT has returned to normal levels. A persisting elevation, up to 2 times the upper normal limit, may herald the onset of chronic hepatitis or cirrhosis, while a continued rise is indicative of massive necrosis and approaching liver failure. Although ALT is elevated in most cases of infectious mononucleosis, peak levels do not exceed 3 times the upper normal limit and gradually fall to normal levels in about 15 weeks. In drug-induced hepatitis, too, the ALT is elevated, often before any other abnormality is found. In contrast, the rise in serum ALT is much more moderate in uncomplicated obstructive jaundice and only when cell necrosis occurs does the enzyme increase dramatically. In this situation the AST/ALT ratio is a rough guide to the extent of cell necrosis. Serum albumin, which is synthesized in the liver, can be a useful indicator of hepatocellular damage. It is somewhat low in this patient, suggesting parenchymal damage, in line with the interpretation of the ALT level.

The role of alkaline phosphatase (AP) in the assessment of jaundice is particularly important. The enzyme has long been known to be present in osteoblasts where it is probably involved in bone mineralization, and when these cells are unusually active, for physiological or pathological reasons, the enzyme appears in the blood. Isoenzyme studies have shown, however, that normally the serum enzyme originates in the liver. Hepatic cells contain one isoenzyme which tends to leak out in moderate amounts in hepatocellular damage; the cells lining the bile canaliculi synthesize another isoenzyme which is excreted in the bile and is, therefore, regurgitated into the blood stream in biliary obstruction. The resulting serum levels of total alkaline phosphatase are often 3–10 times the upper limit of the reference range, according to whether the obstruction is partial or intermittent (stone in bile duct) or complete (e.g., carcinoma). On the other hand, in conditions entailing hepatocellular damage the increases in alkaline phosphatase are not so marked, generally less than 3 times the upper limit. The relatively modest rise manifested on day 2 therefore tends to corroborate the other findings. Subsequently, however, the AP rises steeply, presumably as a result of developing intrahepatic cholestasis to which patients with acute viral hepatitis are prone. The cause of the intrahepatic stasis in these circumstances has not been defined. It may be related to primary damage to the microvilli of the bile canaliculi or to a failure of the bile secretory process of the hepatocyte. The clinical course tends to be prolonged, with more marked and persistent jaundice. The changes in serum enzyme levels in the course of the first 2 weeks highlight the increasing diagnostic complexity as the disease progresses.

On days 7 and 14 the serum bilirubin consists of both conjugated and unconjugated pigment which probably reflects an impaired ability of the liver to carry out the conjugation at this stage. The continued rise in bilirubin and the declining urinary urobilinogen signify an increasing obstruction of bile flow, manifesting also in the pale colour of the faeces. Prothrombin synthesis is deteriorating, either because intestinal absorption of vitamin K is poor in the absence of adequate amounts of bile salts and/or on account of the parenchymal damage to the liver. A shortening of the red cell life span, common in viral hepatitis, is probably responsible for the falling haemoglobin and could contribute to the unconjugated bilirubin in the serum, but the principal cause of the anaemia is probably unconnected with the liver disease and may well be iron deficiency in a young female. The white cell count and distribution remains the same throughout the 3 weeks and hence provides no positive evidence for mononucleosis in which mononuclear cells usually comprise at least 60 per cent of the leucocytes at some stage of the illness.

The third week witnesses a relief of the obstruction: the alkaline phosphatase is declining, the stool colour returns to normal and the prothrombin time is improving, concomitant with a rapid abatement of liver damage suggested by the falling aminotransferase.

On the basis of the available clinical and laboratory evidence we may conclude that the patient has cholestatic viral hepatitis, a benign variant of hepatitis.

Certain investigations should have been done early in the illness, particularly a test for hepatitis B and a careful examination of blood smears for plasmodia and the heterophil agglutination test for mononucleosis. Later on a test for antibody to Epstein-Barr virus would have been indicated, as the EBV is strongly implicated in the aetiology of mononucleosis and can usually be demonstrated.

Needle biopsy of the liver is strongly contraindicated when the clotting time is prolonged. A plain X-ray and other procedures to visualize the gall-bladder and bile duct are probably redundant in the face of good evidence for viral hepatitis with a rapidly subsiding cholestasis. Serum bilirubin and aminotransferase should continue to be monitored until both return to base line, an indication that recovery is complete.

Additional Questions

1. Which of the biochemical data obtained on day 2 would have fitted a diagnosis of glandular fever?
2. If the patient had been black, which condition would have occupied a prominent place in early diagnostic considerations? In what respects might the biochemical data on day 2 have differed?

Further Reading

Mosley, J. W. and Galambos, J. (1975). Viral hepatitis, in *Diseases of the Liver*, ed. Schiff, L., 4th edn., pp. 544–558, J. B. Lippincott Company, Philadelphia.

Case 10

Case History

John H., aged 4, was admitted to hospital with a history of facial oedema for 6–8 weeks. The GP was consulted when periorbital puffiness had persisted for a week and the patient had vomited a few times and had become anorexic. The GP noted leg as well as facial oedema and found the boy's urine to be dark and to contain albumin. Previously the patient's health had been good except for a bout of tonsillitis about 2 months prior to admission.

Examination

The patient was not anaemic or jaundiced. Temperature 36·7 °C.
CVS   Pulse 80 per minute regular.
        Blood pressure 100/70 mm Hg (lying).
        Pitting oedema of ankles.
AS   Liver, kidneys and spleen not palpable. No ascites.
CNS   Trousseau and Chvostek signs positive.
All other systems: no abnormality detected.

Laboratory investigations

Investigation	Result	Reference range
Haemoglobin (g·dl^{-1})	15·6	12 – 14
Red cells (10^{12}. ℓ^{-1})	5·0	4·0 – 5·5
White cells (10^9. ℓ^{-1})	8·8	5 – 15
Serum Na (mmol. ℓ^{-1})	126	132 – 144
Serum K (mmol. ℓ^{-1})	5·2	3·5 – 5·5
Serum Cl (mmol. ℓ^{-1})	92	95 – 105
Serum HCO$_3$ (mmol. ℓ^{-1})	16	24 – 30
Serum phosphate (mmol. ℓ^{-1})	2·18	1·1 – 1·8
Serum urea (mmol. ℓ^{-1})	22·5	2·5 – 7·5
Serum Ca$_{total}$ (mmol. ℓ^{-1})	1·9	2·20 – 2·65
Serum Ca$_{ultrafilterable}$ (mmol. ℓ^{-1})	1·38	1·48 – 1·62
Serum cholesterol (mmol. ℓ^{-1})	17·2	3·6 – 7·2
Serum albumin (g. ℓ^{-1})	10	33 – 48
Serum globulin (g. ℓ^{-1})	26	20 – 37
Serum IgG (IU. ml^{-1})	50	65 – 170
Serum IgA (IU. ℓ^{-1})	13	19 – 112
Serum IgM (IU. ℓ^{-1})	332	50 – 200

Continued on next page

Laboratory Investigations contd

Investigation	Result	Reference range
Urine volume (ml/24h)	150	
Urine protein (mg/h/m^2)	235	<4
Urine creatinine clearance (ml/min/m^2)	31	60 – 90
Urine calcium (mmol/24h)	0·1	2·4 (age 4–12)
Some hyaline casts with fatty inclusions.		

Questions

1. What is the diagnosis?
2. What conclusions can be drawn from the laboratory tests?
3. What treatment would you prescribe? What is the prognosis?

Leading Questions

1. (a) What are the possible causes of oedema and which can be ruled out on the basis of history and examination?
   (b) What are the most common causes of proteinuria?
   (c) Which of the laboratory tests confirm the diagnosis?
   (d) Is there any evidence of a toxin or of a recognizable disease as the causative agent?
   (e) In view of the patient's age is there one particular diagnosis which is the most likely?
2. (a) Several of the serum and urine abnormalities are not directly related to proteinuria. Can they be ascribed to a single pathological circumstance?
   (b) Why did the patient vomit?
   (c) Can you explain why the serum sodium and chloride are low?
   (d) Could undue urinary excretion account for it?
   (e) Why is the total serum calcium low?
   (f) Does the low ionised calcium require a different explanation?
   (g) Which of the factors regulating the serum calcium could account for it?
   (h) How can we explain the Ig levels and what is their clinical significance?
3. (a) Is a specific therapy permissible in this patient without further tests?
   (b) What is the likely course of the illness over the next 12 months?
   (c) How will the treatment relate to this course?

Discussion

In children oedema is usually apparent first in the periorbital area. This boy has generalized oedema by the time of admission which would be evident by a gain in weight (not recorded) as well as by his appearance and examination. In the absence of any detectable abnormalities in the cardiovascular and respiratory systems or in the liver, the nephrotic syndrome is strongly suspected and this is confirmed by the laboratory tests: urinary protein excretion in excess of $40mg.h^{-1}.m^{-2}$, hypoalbuminaemia and generalized oedema define the syndrome. Two other biochemical abnormalities are classically found in the nephrotic syndrome: a low serum calcium and a raised cholesterol.

Proteinuria

Proteinuria of moderate to severe degree is found in many conditions which may be broadly classified into five groups: transient, overflow, glomerular, tubular and nephrogenic (i.e., protein synthesized in the kidney). In the first group are conditions such as exercise, postural and pregnancy proteinurias which are not associated with nephrotic syndrome. Similarly, the amount of protein (e.g., Tamm-Horsfall protein) excreted in the nephrogenic proteinurias is not sufficient to give rise to nephrotic syndrome. High protein excretion on the other hand, is usually associated with glomerular disease and in children 90 per cent are due to primary (idiopathic) glomerulonephritis. A wide variety of diseases, including renal vein thrombosis, Henoch-Schonlein purpura, collagen disorders, drugs and heavy metals, amyloid, post-acute nephritis, malaria, sickle cell disease and allergic nephrosis, give rise to secondary nephrotic syndrome, in several of them due to tubular proteinuria. Low molecular weight proteins (e.g., Bence-Jones protein) are rarely produced in large enough quantities to cause nephrotic syndrome when filtered in normal glomeruli. A small group of children have congenital nephrotic syndrome.

About 80 per cent of children with idiopathic nephrotic syndrome show no evidence of any pathological change in the kidney on light microscopy and the condition is therefore classified as 'minimum change nephropathy' (MCN). Commonly the functional abnormality of the glomerulus in MCN is such as to allow proteins of the molecular size of albumin to pass through while retaining somewhat larger proteins. The size discrimination is roughly quantifiable by means of the 'selectivity index' which is the ratio of IgG and transferrin clearances. The respective molecular weights are 150 000 and 88 000 daltons and an index C_{IgG}/C_{tr} of less than 0·15, often found in MCN, is associated with a good chance of responding to steroids and carries an excellent prognosis. In a child of less than 7 years a high selectivity indicates that the patient is likely to respond to steroids; hence a renal biopsy to establish the diagnosis of MCN is unnecessary.

Plasma calcium

Some of the laboratory data, other than those indicative of the nephrotic syndrome, testify to a degree of renal failure in this case. There is uraemia which accounts for the vomiting; the creatinine clearance is low; the kidney's ability to excrete fixed acids is impaired (metabolic acidosis), and phosphate is retained.

Plasma sodium and chloride are low due to the equilibration of the ions with the expanded tissue fluid and dilution of the plasma by water retention. The factors determining the calcium concentration are more complex. The total serum calcium is always reduced in the nephrotic syndrome because the substantial loss of albumin in the urine lowers the protein-bound fraction. Even so, the physiologically important ionised (or ultrafilterable) fraction in equilibrium with it can often remain within normal limits and would be 1·47 mmol. ℓ^{-1} in this case, but it has fallen to 1·38, which accounts for the positive Trousseau and Chvostek signs. Paradoxically, the urine calcium is also low, due, it is believed, to increased tubular reabsorption of ionic calcium. How then can we explain the hypocalcaemia? As we have seen, there is a degree of renal failure in this patient, but even if hydroxylation of vitamin D were unaffected, much of the vitamin D-binding globulin (MW 58 000, compare with albumin 69 000) together with the active vitamin is lost in the urine. It is, therefore, not surprising that low serum levels of the physiologically active 1,25-dihydroxycholecalciferol (1,25 DHCC) and its precursor 25 HCC have been recorded in the nephrotic syndrome and there are reports of rickets in young children with persistent proteinuria. A failure of calcium absorption normally triggers secondary hyperparathyroidism and so maintains the crucial ionic calcium between narrow limits, but perhaps the response of bone to PTH is depressed in the absence of adequate 1,25 DHCC which is known to have a permissive action. In a remission, when proteinuria diminishes or ceases, the serum calcium quickly returns to normal levels.

Other protein losses

The loss of IgG and IgA in the urine is responsible for the frequency of infections which carried a high mortality before the advent of antibiotics. Other proteins which may be lost in the urine include caeruloplasmin and transferrin, so leading to possible deficiencies of the corresponding cations. Specific globulins binding thyroxine, corticosteroids and vitamin D are also lost in the urine. In the case of thyroxine-binding globulin this leads to a reduction in serum thyroxine and triiodothyronine but TSH and free thyroxine levels are normal and the patient is euthyroid.

Treatment

Treatment consists of prednisolone and diuretics, the latter only to the extent demanded by the patient's state of hydration. It should be recognized that some patients have a reduced plasma volume and that their condition may be aggravated by diuretic therapy. Response to prednisolone is often rapid and leads to substantial amelioration or cessation of proteinuria and concomitant restoration of the serum calcium, both ionic and protein-bound. It may therefore be unnecessary to correct the hypocalcaemia with calcium gluconate. A high protein diet ensures that albumin can be synthesized at an adequate rate but may have to be postponed until renal function has returned to normal. Relapses are common and proteinuria often accompanies even minor infections. In children with MCN the prognosis is excellent: 95 per cent may be expected to make a full recovery.

Pathogenesis

There is little doubt that immunological mechanisms underlie most of the diseases which cause the nephrotic syndrome, be it deposits in the glomeruli of antibody, immune complexes, complement components or coagulation factors. In experimental animals antibodies to the heteropolysaccharides of the glomerular basement membrane cause proteinuria, as do soluble non-glomerular antigens interacting with antibodies to form immuno-complexes which lodge in the glomeruli, damaging the capillaries either directly or by attracting phagocytic cells. Autoantibodies to rheumatoid factor and cryoglobulins have been found in patients with streptococcal infections, SLE and essential cryoglobulinaemia.

In patients who relapse a renal biopsy may be required. Although light microscopy reveals no abnormality of the glomeruli in MCN, in the EM the foot processes are seen to be fused and the coalesced epithelial cytoplasm covers the basement membrane. These changes are present only during active disease manifested by proteinuria: in a remission the foot processes reappear. However it is not clear whether this cellular abnormality is the cause or the consequence of the proteinuria – there is some evidence favouring either notion.

It is commonly believed that loss of protein in the nephrotic syndrome is due to enlarged pores in the basement membrane. Pores cannot be seen under the microscope but measurements of the fractional clearance of uncharged dextrans of various molecular diameters (20–44 Å; albumin 36 Å) have shown that in MCN the pores are actually smaller – about 55 Å compared with the normal size of 59 Å. The reason why albumin passes through glomerular pores in MCN and virtually all other glomerular diseases marked by proteinuria is now known to be a loss of fixed negative charges within the pore, probably dermatan sulphate or sialic acid. It is these fixed charges which normally prevent passage of negatively charged albumin, whereas neutral dextran of the same molecular diameter filters readily. The selectivity index takes no account of charge discrimination which limits its usefulness.

The synthetic capacity of the healthy liver is capable of keeping pace with moderate protein loss in the kidney and one would therefore not expect any hypoproteinaemia. However, a proportion of the protein filtered at the glomerulus is known to be degraded in the tubules and, in addition, some protein may be lost across the intestinal mucosa damaged by oedema. Thus the degree of hypoproteinaemia is often greater than that to be expected from urinary protein loss alone.

Oedema The oedema in nephrotic syndrome is due to hypoalbuminaemia and consequently to the low oncotic pressure of the plasma. Often it is aggravated by sodium retention. There are three potential mechanisms which could account for this phenomenon:

1. The low plasma oncotic pressure and consequent transfer of water into the extracellular fluid and cells leads to hypovolaemia which will lower the glomerular filtration rate and with it the filtration of sodium chloride;
2. Hypovolaemia triggers renin release and hence increased aldosterone secretion which stimulates sodium reabsorption in the distal tubules;

DLDD–F

3. Stimulation of the renal nerve has been shown to result in increased reabsorption of NaCl by the proximal tubules, even in the absence of haemodynamic changes. In this context it should be noted that many patients with MCN do not manifest a reduced plasma volume and they may have normal or lower than normal plasma renin and aldosterone levels. Further, the GFR is usually well maintained. Thus the third mechanism may well be the most usual to account for the salt retention. Nevertheless, the circulation is in a tenuous state which may give rise to renal hypoperfusion, hypotension and uraemia and may be aggravated by interstitial oedema in the kidney itself collapsing renal tubules and restricting glomerular filtration. Together these events undoubtedly are the forerunners of acute renal failure.

Hyperlipidoedema   The hyperlipidaemia which is one of the most striking features of the nephrotic syndrome requires an explanation. Cholesterol, phospholipid and triglyceride levels are all raised in association with the increase in the plasma lipoprotein carriers of these lipids. The low oncotic pressure engendered by the loss of albumin is believed to stimulate hepatic biosynthesis not only of albumin but also of lipoproteins and lipids, since restoration of the osmotic pressure with dextran lowers the plasma lipid level. In addition to increased synthesis of lipoproteins and lipids, catabolism of lipids is reduced, possibly because there is not enough albumin to bind and remove the liberated fatty acids. At the same time some lipid-carrying proteins are filtered at the glomerulus and appear in the urine as fatty acid inclusions.

Additional Questions

1. Why are patients with nephrotic syndrome prone to drug toxicity?
2. Why is hypochromic anaemia sometimes a complication in nephrotic syndrome?

Further Reading

Nephrotic Syndrome, B. M. Brenner & J. H. Stein, eds. Churchill Livingstone, New York, 1982, especially chapter 2, H. J. Reineck, pp. 31–43, chapter 4, D. B. Bernard, pp. 85–114 and chapter 6, J. R. Hoyer, pp. 145–167.

Case 11

Case History

T. H., a 23-year-old trainee solicitor, was admitted to an infectious diseases hospital direct from his home airport. He had become ill on the second day of his holiday in Greece with high fever, vomiting, diarrhoea and abdominal pain. Initially he was treated with antibiotics for several days but he became progressively worse and was transferred home after a short admission to hospital in Greece during which he was given an intravenous infusion. On admission to the ID ward the patient was investigated as a pyrexia of unknown origin (PUO).

Examination

The patient was restless, uncooperative and in some pain. He had a maculopapular rash over the arms and buttocks. The left elbow was inflamed at the site of the IV infusion. There was no anaemia, jaundice or lymphadenopathy. Temperature 39.5 °C.

CVS Pulse 120 per minute regular.
     Blood pressure 130/70 mm Hg (lying).
     Hearts sounds normal.
RS   Respiratory rate 28 per minute.
     Chest clear.
AS   Mild generalized tenderness.
     Liver, kidneys and spleen not felt.
     No other masses palpable.
CNS Normal.
MSS Mild generalized muscle tenderness.

Progress

Over ten days the patient became more difficult to manage. He was reluctant to sit up in bed or stand and vomited his food 3–4 times daily. The nursing staff described him as extremely difficult and uncooperative. Investigation of his PUO produced uniformly negative results, but he was treated empirically with further courses of antibiotics. As he had become incapable of taking oral nutrition or fluid a course of IV nutrition was commenced on the tenth day. An estimation of serum calcium prior to starting his IV nutrition revealed severe hypercalcaemia. Examination at that time showed the patient was hypotensive with a blood pressure of 90/70 mm Hg (lying) which dropped even further on standing.

Laboratory investigations

Investigation	Result On admission	Day 7	Day 10	Reference range
Plasma sodium (mmol. ℓ^{-1})	120	130	125	135 – 145
Plasma potassium (mmol. ℓ^{-1})	3·8	5·0	5·4	3·5 – 5·3
Plasma chloride (mmol. ℓ^{-1})	78	92	89	98 – 108
Plasma bicarbonate (mmol. ℓ^{-1})	20		16	22 – 30
Plasma urea (mmol. ℓ^{-1})	12·1	7·0	11·2	2·5 – 7·5
Plasma osmolality (mmol. kg^{-1})			270	275 – 295
Serum bilirubin (μmol. ℓ^{-1})	20		25	<17
Serum alanine aminotransferase (IU. ℓ^{-1})	30		70	15 – 55
Serum total protein (g. ℓ^{-1})	65		66	62 – 82
Serum albumin (g. ℓ^{-1})	32		35	37 – 47
Serum alkaline phosphatase (IU. ℓ^{-1})	125		140	30 – 110
Serum calcium (mmol. ℓ^{-1})	2·24[a]		3·05	2·25 – 2·65
Serum phosphate (mmol. ℓ^{-1})			1·81	1·1 – 1·8
Serum urate (mmol. ℓ^{-1})			0·53	0·18 – 0·48
Serum creatinine phosphokinase (IU. ℓ^{-1})			86	25 – 190
Blood glucose (mmol. ℓ^{-1}) (fasting)	4·9			2·5 – 5·0
Urine osmolality (mmol. kg^{-1})			452	500 – 800[b]
Creatinine clearance (ml. min^{-1})			55	90 – 130

[a] Calcium determined on a serum specimen obtained on the day of admission and stored for virology. Analysis carried out on day 15.
[b] On normal fluid intake. Potential range 50–1400 mmol. kg^{-1}.

Questions

1. What is the differential diagnosis on the tenth day of his admission?
2. How can the most likely diagnosis be confirmed with biochemical and other investigations?
3. What treatment should be given and how should this be monitored?

Leading Questions

1. (a) What are the most informative biochemical abnormalities on day 10?
   (b) Can any additional information be obtained from the specimens taken on days 1 and 7?
   (c) What diagnoses are suggested by:
      (i) the hypercalcaemia,
      (ii) the electrolyte abnormalities?
   (d) Do the clinical observations contradict or support any of these diagnoses?
   (e) Is there a single diagnosis which could encompass the electrolyte and calcium abnormalities?
   (f) Do the biochemical changes account wholly, or in part, for the patient's signs and symptoms?
2. (a) What is the main organ system affected, what is its physiological role and how is this controlled?
   (b) What pathological processes can cause a reduction in the activity of that organ?
   (c) What are the common biochemical consequences of these different pathologies?
   (d) How may the function of the organ be directly assessed by pharmacological means?
   (e) Will the results of tests differ according to the aetiology of the disease?
   (f) Can alteration in the activity of the affected organ be iatrogenic? How could assessment of organ function be undertaken in these circumstances?
   (g) What other non-biochemical investigations should be carried out in this patient?
3. (a) What are the objectives of treatment?
   (b) Which physiological compounds will need to be replaced in this patient?
   (c) Is there any value in varying the dosage throughout the day?
   (d) How can the effectiveness of the dose be controlled for each compound?
   (e) What are the signs, symptoms and biochemical changes observed in over and underdosage?

Discussion

After the patient's admission to the infectious diseases ward the pursuit of a cause for the PUO had led to the low plasma sodium and chloride in the initial investigations being attributed to vomiting and IV therapy. As the patient had been abroad, infective causes were high on the list of possible diagnoses but a wide variety of tests for common and obscure bacterial and viral aetiologies were all negative. In particular typhoid was excluded. Hepatitis A or B were unlikely in view of the short period of time before the patient became ill although he could have become infected with hepatitis virus or other agent before leaving for Greece.

The psychiatric disturbances manifested by the patient were initially put down to personality problems though there was little evidence to back this up. His behaviour was volatile and he complained of many symptoms. Possibly these manifestations could have been due to hyperpyrexia but in fact the patient's temperature had never risen above 38.5 °C after admission and fell slowly throughout the first week of his stay. A metabolic cause for his psychosis therefore seemed likely.

Significance of hypercalcaemia

When, on day 10, hypercalcaemia was unexpectedly discovered it provided a convincing explanation of many of the patient's symptoms including nausea, vomiting, fatigue, confusion and increased sensitivity to pain. Preoccupation with the cause of the PUO then gave way to a reappraisal of the earlier findings and a re-examination of the electrolytes. Calcium was determined on day 15 in the serum specimen taken on admission and stored for virological studies: it was found to be normal at 2.24 mmol. ℓ^{-1} which showed that it had risen to hypercalcaemic levels during the first ten days and thus represented an aggravation rather than the cause of the original condition. The hyponatraemia, evident from the day of admission, had been accompanied by increasing plasma potassium concentrations over the next 10 days. The most likely explanation now seemed to be adrenal insufficiency but renal damage secondary to other conditions had to be considered as a cause of the electrolyte abnormality.

Although hypercalcaemia is associated with Addison's disease and so would be in accord with this explanation for the hyponatraemia and hyperkalaemia, it must be remembered that 90 per cent of adult cases of hypercalcaemia are due to primary hyperparathyroidism or skeletal malignancy, both of which increase bone resorption. In the light of the elevated serum phosphate and only moderately compromised renal function the former can be excluded. Malignancy is unlikely at the age of 23 but it can not be entirely discounted in view of the slightly raised alkaline phosphatase. Rarer causes of hypercalcaemia from increased bone resorption are immobilization and thyrotoxicosis, while vitamin D overdose, tuberculosis and sarcoidosis have a similar effect by increasing calcium absorption from the gut. Finally hypercalcaemia is associated with various other diseases including familial hypocalciuric hypercalcaemia and acute renal failure under treatment with thiazide diuretics.

Other electrolyte changes

The patient's poor fluid intake and retention accounts for his dehydration, indicated by the moderately elevated plasma urea, which excludes haemodilution as a cause of the hyponatraemia. Equally salt wasting associated with chronic renal failure can be excluded by the creatinine clearance which is not greatly reduced. The syndrome of inappropriate ADH secretion is also excluded by the mildly elevated plasma urea as well as the increase in serum urate. On balance, therefore, the electrolyte changes are most probably the result of adrenocortical insufficiency, with a lack of mineralocorticoid activity leading to a loss of sodium in the urine and retention of potassium and hydrogen ion.

Investigation of adrenocortical insufficiency

The specific diagnosis of adrenocortical insufficiency is made by measurement of the response of the adrenal glands to synthetic ACTH (Synacthen, α-1-24 tetracosactrin). A dose of 250 μg Synacthen is given IV or IM and cortisol concentrations are measured in plasma at the time of injection and 30 minutes later. The 30 minute value should be at least 200 nmol. ℓ^{-1} above basal and reach an absolute value of 550 nmol. ℓ^{-1} for a normal response. (NB These values may vary between laboratories and are for guidance only). In the patient the basal and peak values were <10 and 10 nmol. ℓ^{-1} respectively.

Adrenal failure can either be primary due to some structural or functional abnormality of the adrenal gland or secondary as a result of hypothalamic-pituitary disease or previous treatment with glucocorticoids. Extremely rarely peripheral insensitivity to glucocorticoids can give rise to a clinical picture of adrenal failure. Differentiation of primary from secondary adrenal insufficiency is made on the basis of a prolonged stimulation of the adrenal glands in which depot Synacthen is given IM on each of 3 days. Plasma cortisol is measured 5 hours after each injection: patients with secondary adrenal insufficiency will show a substantial rise in cortisol concentration. The result of the 3 day Synacthen test on T.H. showed a basal plasma cortisol level of 23 nmol. ℓ^{-1} and a complete lack of response confirming primary adrenal failure. Occasionally patients who have adrenal insufficiency due to partial pituitary suppression following prolonged therapeutic use of glucocorticoids may show a normal response to exogenous ACTH. This group of patients may be studied using tests which evaluate the complete hypothalamic-pituitary-adrenal axis, e.g., the insulin stress and metyrapone tests. In the former insulin-induced hypoglycaemia causes the release of ACTH and stimulation of cortisol synthesis and release. For the test to be valid, effective hypoglycaemia (<2.3 mmol. ℓ^{-1}) must be achieved. There are obvious dangers in this test of inducing hypoglycaemic coma with consequent neurological sequelae or even death, particularly if adrenal function is compromised. The principle of the metyrapone test is to interrupt the feedback control of ACTH release by cortisol. The drug inhibits cortisol synthesis at the 11-hydroxylation step; the accumulation of the precursor 11-deoxycortisol can be measured. Patients with hypothalamic or pituitary disorders will fail to produce cortisol in response to hypoglycaemia and in the metapyrone test will not manifest a rise in 11-deoxycortisol despite the removal of feedback inhibition of ACTH release. Direct measurement of ACTH, when available, is an obvious way of differentiating between primary and secondary adrenal insufficiency. It is important to remember the circadian rhythm of ACTH secretion and take the blood sample at 09.00 hours. Plasma ACTH concentration in this patient was high at 235 ng. ℓ^{-1} (normal 09.00 hours value 10–80 ng. ℓ^{-1}).

Aetiology

Having established the diagnosis of primary adrenal failure in this patient, there remains the problem of the exact aetiology. Additional tests should include radiology for adrenal calcification, autoantibodies to adrenal and other endocrine glands and tests for tuberculosis and sarcoidosis. These tests were all negative in this patient. Other rare causes of adrenal insufficiency, e.g., congenital adrenal hyperplasia usually present in childhood, often in the neonatal period, but cases of congenital adrenal hyperplasia have been identified in adults as a result of HLA typing in affected families and subsequently confirmed with the appropriate biochemical tests, e.g., plasma 17α-hydroxyprogesterone.

Therapy

Treatment of adrenocortical failure is by replacement therapy but primary resuscitative measures are needed in adrenal crisis with the administration of saline and glucose. Hypoglycaemia is often observed in adrenal failure, glucocorticoids being insulin antagonists as well as promoting gluconeogenesis. Steroid replacement with glucocorticoid is given in divided doses with approximately two thirds in the morning to mimic the natural circadian rhythm. One of the objectives of replacement is to inhibit ACTH secretion and the consequent hyperpigmentation. This may require the higher dose of glucocorticoid to be given in the evening. The natural hormone cortisol can be used but alternatively synthetic glucocorticoids such as prednisolone with longer plasma half lives may have some advantage in keeping the pituitary suppressed. Patients with primary adrenal failure will usually require in addition a mineralocorticoid and as the natural hormone aldosterone is unsuitable for oral administration, the synthetic derivative fludrocortisone is used. This drug need only be given once a day. Control of both glucocorticoid and mineralocorticoid replacement relies on clinical examination, e.g., for increasing pigmentation, hypertension or hypotension and Cushingoid features and biochemical assessment of plasma electrolytes. In difficult cases plasma renin estimations are of value; these should be in the normal range if replacement mineralocorticoid is adequate.

Some of the causes of adrenal failure are genetic or familial and questions concerning the medical history of relatives are important. The most common cause is auto-immune adrenal disease with destruction of the adrenal cortex but preservation of the medulla. These patients often have circulating autoantibodies to the adrenal and frequently to other endocrine glands. Autoantibodies were not found in this patient, neither was any evidence of other causes of adrenal failure, e.g., tuberculosis and malignancy. The aetiology of the adrenal failure in this patient remains obscure.

Hypercalcaemia and Addisons' disease

The cause of the hypercalcaemia found in association with Addisons's disease is not known. There are two hypotheses. It has been suggested that in Addison's disease there is an increase of bone resorption resulting from an increased sensitivity to vitamin D and causing hypercalcaemia. The alternative hypothesis is that the decreased glucocorticoid concentrations cause a contraction in ECF and enhanced reabsorption of calcium. This would lead to hypercalcaemia and under normal circumstances compensatory reductions in calcium absorption from the gut and bone resorption would restore the serum calcium to normal. Therefore if this hypothesis is true the homeostatic regulation of calcium must also be functionally inadequate. There is no evidence for either hypothesis.

Additional Questions

1. Explain the patient's acidosis.
2. These patients often have nocturia. Why is this?

Further Reading

Irvine, W. J. and Barnes, E. W. (1972) Adrenocortical insufficiency. *Clin. Endocrinol. Metab.* **1**, pp. 549–594.
Pedersen, K. O. (1967) Hypercalcaemia in Addison's disease. *Acta Med. Scand.* **181**, pp. 691–698.

Case 12

Case History

J. S., a 60-year-old lorry driver, was a known asthmatic who was successfully controlled on cromoglycate. Six weeks prior to admission he had a sudden attack of severe pain in the lower thoracic spine which began when he attempted to lift a heavy object onto his lorry. X-rays of his chest and spine at that time showed no obvious abnormality. Two weeks later he began to have pain in his ribs, right upper arm and both knees. His speech became slightly slurred.

On questioning he revealed that he had nocturia 2–3 times but with a good stream, occasional upper abdominal pain and mild diarrhoea. In the past he had been investigated for a duodenal ulcer which was treated medically. He was a non-smoker and drank only moderate amounts of alcohol. His appetite was good and his weight had not changed.

Examination

The patient was very pale with obvious clinical anaemia. There was no jaundice. Temperature 37 °C.

CVS   Pulse 88 per minute regular.
      Blood pressure 110/70 mm Hg (lying).
      Heart sounds normal.
      No signs of heart failure.
RS   Chest clinically clear.
AS   Some tenderness in the epigastric region.
      PR normal.
CNS   Some slurring of speech.
      Reflexes difficult to elicit.

Laboratory investigations

On admission

Investigation	Result	Reference range
Plasma sodium (mmol. ℓ^{-1})	137	135–145
Plasma potassium (mmol. ℓ^{-1})	3·7	3·5–5·5
Plasma chloride (mmol. ℓ^{-1})	108	98–108

Continued on next page

Laboratory Investigations contd

Investigation	Result	Reference range
Plasma bicarbonate (mmol. ℓ^{-1})	26	22–30
Plasma urea (mmol. ℓ^{-1})	9·8	2·5–7·5
Plasma anion gap (mmol. ℓ^{-1})	7·3	12–18
Serum calcium (mmol. ℓ^{-1})	2·32	2·25–2·65
Serum phosphate (mmol. ℓ^{-1})	1·52	0·8–1·6
Serum urate (mmol. ℓ^{-1})	0·57	0·17–0·48
Serum protein (g. ℓ^{-1})	54	62–82
Serum albumin (g. ℓ^{-1})	35	35–50
Alkaline phosphatase (IU. ℓ^{-1})	80	30–110
Alanine aminotransferase (IU. ℓ^{-1})	16	15–55
Serum iron (μmol. ℓ^{-1})	25	13–32
TIBC (μmol. ℓ^{-1})	41	45–72
Hæmoglobin (g. dl^{-1})	7·9	13–17
RBC ($\times 10^{12}$. ℓ)	2·57	4·5–6·5
PCV (1. ℓ^{-1})	0·25	0·40–0·49
MCHC (g. dl^{-1})	32	31–35
MCV (fl)	97	80–92
MCH (pg)	31	27–32
WBC ($\times 10^9$. ℓ^{-1})	3·7	4·0–11
Platelets ($\times 10^9$. ℓ^{-1})	275	150–400
ESR (mm. h^{-1})	28	<15
White cell differential	normal	
Creatinine clearance (ml. min^{-1})	47	78–147
Proteinuria	+++	negative
Urine culture	negative	
Faecal occult blood	negative ×3	

Later investigations

Serum and urine electrophoresis: a discrete M-band or paraprotein in the gamma region with almost total absence of normal immuno-globulins was observed in serum. An identical band was present in the electrophoresis of unconcentrated urine.

Investigation	Result	Reference range
Serum IgA (g. ℓ^{-1})	<0·4	0·53–4·8
Serum IgG (g. ℓ^{-1})	4·5	6·6–19
Serum IgM (g. ℓ^{-1})	<0·3	0·4–18
Urine total protein (g. $24h^{-1}$)	30·3	<0·15
Urine λ light chains (g. $24h^{-1}$)	24·4	not detected
Urine κ light chains (mg. $24h^{-1}$)	4·0	not detected

Bone marrow aspirate: 35 per cent plasma cells. (Normal <15 per cent).

Questions

1. What is the clinical differential diagnosis at the time of onset of the first symptoms and at the time of admission?
2. What information can be obtained from the initial laboratory investigations on admission?
3. How would you investigate this patient further?

Leading Questions

1. (a) What are the causes of acute back pain?
   (b) Are there any predisposing factors in this patient?
   (c) Do the X-ray findings assist in narrowing the differential diagnosis?
   (d) Which diagnoses are supported by the symptoms of bone pain, nocturia and slurred speech?
   (e) Is the information obtained from the clinical examination of diagnostic value?
2. (a) What are the abnormal biochemical findings in this patient on admission?
   (b) Does involvement of any particular organ system(s) in the disease process suggest a possible approach to diagnosis?
   (c) How is proteinuria usually detected? Are there any defects in this method?
   (d) What alternative and additional methods should be used to examine the urinary protein both qualitatively and quantitatively?
   (e) Is there any diagnostic significance in the electrolyte results?
   (f) What are the abnormal haematological findings?
   (g) Does the history suggest a likely cause for anaemia?
   (h) What factors can modify the ESR?
3. (a) Having identified the nature of the urinary protein as Bence–Jones protein, what further investigations would you undertake?
   (b) What is the source of Bence–Jones protein?
   (c) Why can estimation of total serum protein be misleading in the investigation of patients with this condition?
   (d) Is there any prognostic significance in identifying the type of abnormal paraprotein and/or Bence–Jones protein?
   (e) How can calcium homeostasis be affected in myeloma patients?
   (f) What complication associated with the deposition of extracellular protein can occur in these patients?

Discussion

Acute onset of severe back pain on straining would suggest vertebral collapse from osteoporosis, neoplastic or infectious causes, slipped intervertebral disc or injury to ligaments, muscles or joints. The initial X-rays in this patient would appear to exclude vertebral collapse and make the diagnosis of a disc lesion unlikely. The later symptoms of more generalized bone pain, renal symptoms (nocturia) and neurological abnormalities (slurring of speech) indicate that the disease is a multisystem one. At this patient's age the most likely explanation for all these symptoms is malignancy. Apart from the severe anaemia the clinical examination was not helpful. The patient was a non-smoker and the first chest X-ray did not show evidence of lung pathology.

Initial biochemical investigation on admission showed several abnormal results: urea, phosphate and uric acid were all raised while the total protein was low. A normal alkaline phosphatase reduces the likelihood of secondary carcinomatosis involving the bones. Creatinine clearance was reduced and there was a considerable quantity of protein in the urine. The haematological investigations showed a severe anaemia, which was normochromic with some macrocytosis. With a past history of duodenal ulcer and a possible gastrointestinal malignancy, loss of blood from the gut was excluded by the negative occult blood, normal serum iron and TIBC. None of the results from these investigations give rise to a specific diagnosis but the reduced renal function together with heavy proteinuria would indicate a useful line of further investigation. If the patient has a neoplasm then this could either be of primary renal origin with secondary spread or the kidneys could themselves be affected secondarily by a malignant process elsewhere. By identifying the nature of the urine protein the differential diagnosis is considerably narrowed.

Urine protein

Screening for urine protein is usually with Albustix or some other dipstick procedure. These methods can, as in this case, considerably underestimate actual protein excretion when the major protein is not albumin. Better assessment of proteinuria can be made with sulphosalicylic acid precipitation which can be developed into a quantitative test. Although Bence–Jones protein can be identified by simple techniques, these screening tests can give rise to false negative results. More definitive identification of urine protein requires electrophoresis (usually after considerable concentration of the urine) and immunoelectrophoresis. In this patient there was so much protein in the urine that concentration was unnecessary; indeed dilution was required for the classical heat solubility test for Bence–Jones protein. All tests identified the major protein excreted as Bence–Jones protein. It is identical with the light chain of immunoglobulin and with a molecular weight of 22 000 daltons (44 000 when dimeric) is easily filtered at the glomerulus and cleared from plasma; thus Bence–Jones protein is only present in plasma when there is renal failure. Light chains are found in urine in several different disorders of the immunocyte but is most common in myeloma. Other causes include soft tissue plasmacytoma, Waldenstrom's macroglobulinaemia, non-Hodgkins lymphoma and chronic lymphatic leukaemia.

Significance of serum protein

The further investigation of Bence–Jones proteinuria requires the examination of the serum proteins by electrophoresis together with measurement of the individual immunoglobulins, a bone marrow aspiration and a skeletal survey. The results of these investigations showed a faint monoclonal band (M-band) on the electrophoresis with a reduction in all the three major subgroups of the immuno-globulins (immunoparesis), a large increase in marrow plasma cells and lytic lesions in the skull, pelvis, ribs and humeri. These classical findings are conclusive for the diagnosis of myeloma. Lytic lesions in the bones are caused by local plasma cell accumulation. Back pain is a frequent presenting symptom in myeloma but vertebral lesions may be absent on X-ray.

Plasma cells are the major source of the circulating immuno-globulins and are the terminal stage in the maturation of the B-series lymphocytes. Each cell normally produces only one specific antibody of a single immunoglobulin class (IgG, IgA, IgM, IgD and IgE) with the appropriate heavy chain (γ, α, μ, δ and ϵ) and only one type of light chain (κ and λ). When a plasma cell becomes malignant it multiplies and the balance between the synthesis of heavy and light chains can be disturbed, usually with the production of excess light chain. In 80 per cent of myelomas a monoclonal immuno-globulin appears in the plasma and two-thirds of these will produce excess light chain excreted in the urine as Bence–Jones protein. The monoclonal protein is usually either an IgG or an IgA immunoglobulin. In almost all the remaining 20 per cent dedifferentiation has progressed to the point that only light chains are produced. A small number of patients will have IgD, IgM or IgE myelomas, occasionally two M-bands may be found or the plasma cell can be non-secretory. Identification and quantification of the M-band and the light chain type of Bence–Jones protein is performed by immunochemical and immunoelectrophoretic methods. The identification of the light chain type is of particular importance as the prognosis of the kappa excretor is poorer. Quantification of the M-band and Bence–Jones protein is useful in monitoring therapy. Total serum protein measurement in myeloma is highly variable and depends not only on the quantity of the paraprotein but also on the reduction in the normal immunoglobulins and, late in the disease, in albumin. In this patient the total serum protein was low at diagnosis in the presence of a normal albumin.

Some effects of paraprotein

Patients with myeloma may exhibit several abnormalities in biochemical and haematological investigations. A few of these are brought about primarily because of the presence of the paraprotein in the plasma. The patients usually have a high ESR due to alteration in the albumin/globulin ratio and increased rouleaux formation. The latter can give rise to a spuriously increased MCV and apparent macrocytosis. True macrocytosis associated with folate deficiency is found in 10 per cent of myeloma patients. Hyperviscosity due to the quantity and type of paraprotein can lead to neurological and other symptoms. The paraprotein is often cationic (i.e., positively charged) at physiological pH which narrows the anion gap due to obligatory retention of chloride and bicarbonate. An anion gap of <10 mmol. ℓ^{-1} (normal 12–18 mmol. ℓ^{-1}) is found in 30 per cent of myeloma patients and this can be a clue to the presence of the disease. The anion gap in J. S. was 7·3 mmol. ℓ^{-1}. Patients with a large concentration of paraprotein in the plasma can show spurious hyponatraemia (Case No. 18) and this hyponatraemia will exacerbate the low anion gap.

Other biochemical abnormalities frequently found include hypercalcaemia often related to skeletal involvement and more severe in can bind calcium which can cause or exacerbate hypercalcaemia. Alkaline phosphatase is usually normal in the absence of fractures, probably due to the lack of osteoblastic activity associated with bony plasma cell tumours. Renal function is often impaired with increased plasma urea and serum creatinine, phosphate and uric acid, due to the formation of light chain casts which cause a cellular reaction leading to progressive tubular atrophy. Renal failure can occur in IgA myeloma in the absence of Bence–Jones proteinuria. The presence of hypercalcaemia and dehydration can exacerbate the renal impairment. Uric acid can rise considerably during therapy due to the destruction of the malignant cells and give rise to gout.

Amyloid

Amyloid deposits are found in the kidneys and other tissues of 10 per cent of patients. In the amyloid associated with myeloma and other B-cell tumours the major protein is identical with the variable portion of the monoclonal light chain and is highly resistant to physiological or pharmacological attempts to remove it. A minor component present in all types of amyloid, both primary and secondary, is the P component which has an unusual pentameric structure and is an acute phase reactant. Another plasma protein Amyloid A (AA) protein is the major component in most types of secondary amyloid.

Serum paraproteins can be found in a number of conditions other than myeloma and together account for 40 per cent of all paraproteins. The more common conditions include Waldenstroms macroglobulinaemia, soft tissue plasmacytoma and lymphosarcoma. Approximately half of the non-myeloma paraproteins are referred to as benign paraproteins or monoclonal gammopathy of unknown significance. In contradistinction to myeloma immunoglobulin fragments are rarely if ever found. Normal immunoglobulins are present on electrophoresis of serum. Paraprotein levels are mostly < 1g. ℓ^{-1} and the concentration remains stable over a considerable number of years without treatment. A number of these patients do, however develop myeloma, macroglobulinaemia, amyloid or lymphoma after a long latent period and all patients should be followed.

Additional Questions

1. What immunological activity has been associated with monoclonal myeloma proteins?
2. What are the clinical consequences of amyloid?

Further Reading

Whicher, J. T. (1983). Abnormalities of Plasma Proteins. In Scientific Foundation of Clinical Biochemistry: *Biochemistry in Clinical Practice*. Eds Williams, D. L. and Marks, V. pp. 221–251 Heinemann Medical Books, London.

Glenner, G. G. (1980) Amyloid Deposits and Amyloidosis. *New Engl. J. Med.*, **302**, pp. 1283–1292 and 1333–1343.

Case 13

Case History

Robert L., a 25-year-old postman, was seen at the arthritis clinic at the request of his GP whom the patient had consulted a few times over the past 3 years for pain in the right Achilles tendon. Attacks seemed to occur several times a year, particularly after physical exertion, and last 3 or 4 days, with the pain becoming so intense that he could not continue on his round, only to subside gradually over the next few days. Occasionally both Achilles tendons and knees were affected. The GP had prescribed aspirin and later indomethacin, but attacks had continued.

Examination

During an attack both Achilles tendons were found to be oedematous, inflamed and tender to palpation. Pain was exacerbated by dorsiflexing the foot. Knees were swollen and erythematous. Xanthomas were noted over both Achilles tendons and over the extensor tendons of the hands. Temperature 36.2 °C.
All other systems: no abnormality detected.
X-ray of ankles and knees normal.

Laboratory investigations

Investigation	Result	Reference Range
Haemoglobin (g/dl)	14·0	13·0 – 17·0
Red blood cells ($10^{12}.\ell^{-1}$)	5·2	4·2 – 6·5
White blood cells ($10^9.\ell^{-1}$)	5·6	4·0 – 11·0
ESR (mm. h^{-1})	10	0 – 12
Blood smear: no abnormal cells.		
Plasma Na (mmol. ℓ^{-1})	138	135 – 145
Plasma K (mmol. ℓ^{-1})	3·6	3·3 – 5·3
Serum total protein (g. ℓ^{-1})	64	62 – 82
Serum albumin (g. ℓ^{-1})	40	35 – 50
Serum Ca (mmol. ℓ^{-1})	2·3	2·25 – 2·75
Serum phosphate (mmol. ℓ^{-1})	1·4	0·8 – 1·6
Serum alkaline phosphatase (IU. ℓ^{-1})	80	30 – 110
Serum urea (mmol. ℓ^{-1})	4·1	2·5 – 7·5
Serum glucose (mmol. ℓ^{-1})	4·2[a]	3·0 – 5·3
Serum uric acid (mmol. ℓ^{-1})	0·35	0·17 – 0·48

Continued on next page

Laboratory Investigations contd

Investigation	Result	Reference range
Serum cholesterol (mmol. ℓ^{-1})	$9{\cdot}0^a$	$4{\cdot}5-6{\cdot}5$
Serum triglycerides (mmol. ℓ^{-1})	$1{\cdot}6^a$	$0{\cdot}7-2{\cdot}1$
Urine protein	0	0
Lipoprotein electrophoresis	increased lipoprotein.	
Serum	clear	

[a] After overnight fast.

Questions

1. What is the diagnosis?
2. What is the aetiology of the condition?
3. Is there a specific therapy?

Leading Questions

1. (a) Which diagnostic possibilities suggested by the patient's symptoms can be eliminated on the basis of the biochemical profile?
   (b) Hypercholesterolaemia may be primary or secondary. What are the conditions giving rise to it? Which of them are unlikely in the light of the patient's history and the result of laboratory investigations?
   (c) What are xanthomas?
   (d) Is their presence in accord with the laboratory findings?
   (e) Is there a single diagnosis which accounts for all facts elucidated so far?
   (f) Is the condition hereditary?
   (g) Would you expect investigations of the patient's close relatives to be helpful?
2. (a) What are the sources of plasma cholesterol?
   (b) What are the functions of cholesterol in the liver, endocrine glands and peripheral tissues?
   (c) How is cholesterol transported in the plasma?
   (d) How does plasma cholesterol get into the cells and what role does the transport protein play in this mechanism?
   (e) Do cells require special equipment for this mechanism to function?
   (f) Do you know any diseases in which this type of equipment is faulty?

(g) Can the plasma cholesterol be lowered by dietary measures or by altering intestinal function?

(h) What is the rate-determining step in cholesterol biosynthesis and how could it be inhibited?

Discussion

The patient presents with some symptoms suggestive of arthritis and its commonly associated tenosynovitis. A normal serum urate makes gout unlikely as a precipitating factor of his arthritic condition. Systemic lupus erythematosus (SLE) is unlikely in view of the normal temperature and ESR, as well as the absence of specific LE cells in the blood smear. The single abnormality in his biochemical investigation is the serum cholesterol, although the definition of normal limits is inevitably arbitrary and values vary with age, sex and even the geographical location. Ideally, the lipids are measured in the form in which they are transported in the blood, i.e., in association with apoproteins, but separation of lipoproteins by analytical centrifugation is time-consuming and quantitative electrophoresis suffers from lack of proper standards. For everyday purposes visual examination of fasting plasma for lipaemia and chylomicrons, qualitative electrophoresis for lipoproteins, together with determination of total cholesterol and triglycerides is the most commonly used procedure.

Hypercholesterolaemia

The cholesterol is carried mainly (70 per cent) in the form of low density lipoprotein (LDL) and thus an increase in that fraction usually results in hypercholesterolaemia. In contrast, triglycerides are largely associated with the lighter particles – chylomicrons and very low density lipoproteins (VLDL) – on which they confer the low density. In this patient the hypercholesterolaemia signifies an increased plasma concentration of LDL, while the normal triglyceride level indicates that there is no generalised hyperlipidaemia.

The common primary hyperlipoproteinaemias have been classified according to the particular plasma lipoprotein which is elevated. All have a familial incidence (*Table 13.1*).

Hypercholesterolaemia is a common sequela of a variety of conditions, including biliary obstruction, diabetes, nephrotic syndrome and hypothyroidism. There is no evidence of any of these in the patient and primary or familial hypercholesterolaemia must therefore be considered. Type II (hyper β) lipoproteinaemia manifests in the majority of patients with raised plasma cholesterol. It includes familial hyperlipoproteinaemia (FH), with an autosomal dominant inheritance and an incidence of the heterozygous state of 1:500, and

Table 13.1 Classification of primary hyperlipoproteinaemias

Elevated plasma lipoprotein	Major form of disease	Type
Chylomicrons	Lipoprotein lipase deficiency	I
VLDL	Hypertriglyceridaemia (mild)	IV
VLDL + chylomicrons	Hypertriglyceridaemia (severe)	V
LDL	Hypercholesterolaemia	IIa
LDL + VLDL	Multiple lipoprotein-type hyperlipidaemia	IIb
β VLDL	Dysbetalipoproteinaemia	III

the less clearly defined but more common condition of polygenic hypercholesterolaemia. Questioning and laboratory investigation of first degree relatives should therefore provides a valuable clue to the diagnosis, for the triad of familial incidence, hypercholesterolaemia and tendon xanthoma is virtually pathognomonic for FH. In Type III hyperlipoproteinaemia abnormally large amounts of cholesterol are associated with triglycerides in VLDL and result in approximately equal, raised, levels of the two lipids, unless the triglycerides exceed $5 - 10$ mmol. ℓ^{-1}.

The patient's xanthomas are nodular swellings of tendons of the dorsum of the hand, elbow, knee and ankle formed by deposition in interstitial spaces of macrophages laden with cholesterol esters. Cholesterol is often deposited also in the eyelids and within the cornea, constituting xanthelasma and arcus lipoides corneae respectively. Unlike xanthomas over tendons, the latter are not typical of familial hypercholesterolaemia.

LDL Receptor

FH results from one of several genetic defects in a cell surface receptor which normally controls the endocytosis and hence the metabolism of LDL. Heterozygotes for the disease are hypercholesterolaemic from birth, although they often remain asymptomatic until the third or fourth decade, when xanthomas develop in tendons and other sites and atheroma in arteries. Myocardial infarction in that age group is thus more common in heterozygotes than in the general population. By age 60 years 85 per cent of heterozygotes have had a myocardial infarct.

Of the two alleles responsible for the heterozygous state, one codes for normal receptor protein while the other codes for an abnormal and probably non-functional protein. Thus the patient is endowed with only one half of the usual density of functioning receptors on the cell surface, which impairs his ability to endocytose LDL. Homozygotes for FH have a double dose of the abnormal allele. They and the more numerous patients who have two different genes, both of which are abnormal, are totally unable to absorb LDL into their cells. In these individuals death from myocardial infarction in childhood is not uncommon. Patients with a single as well as a double dose of abnormal alleles may have recurrent polyarthritis and tenosynovitis.

Origin and transport of cholesterol

There are two sources of plasma cholesterol: the diet and synthesis *de novo*, mainly in the liver. The committed step in the biosynthesis is the formation of mevalonic acid from 3-hydroxy-3-methylglutaryl CoA, catalyzed by a reductase which regulates the over-all process. In fact, the synthesis of this enzyme is inhibited by cholesterol, irrespective of the sterol's source. Thus it is important to bear in mind that dietary cholesterol is a potent inhibitor of endogenous synthesis.

Cholesterol is transported in the plasma in association with specific apoproteins, especially apoprotein B in LDL, which serve to solubilize the water-insoluble lipids. The liver synthesizes VLDL, containing triglycerides as well as cholesterol esters, primarily for delivery of the former to adipose tissue. After disposal of triglycerides and some of the apoproteins, the residue containing mainly apoprotein B and cholesterol esters, constitutes LDL whose role it is to transport cholesterol and ensure its uptake by the tissues for incorporation into their membranes and for storage. Specific receptors on the plasma membrane of non-hepatic cells, located in special regions termed 'coated pits', recognize lipoprotein B and form receptor-LDL complexes which are then internalized by invagination and formation of an endocytic vesicle. Once within the cell, the vesicle fuses with lysosomes whose enzymes hydrolyze apo-B to amino acids and the cholesterol ester to free cholesterol which is then either incorporated into the lipid bilayer or re-esterified to a special storage ester.

Regulation of cholesterol synthesis and disposal

The cholesterol content of the cell exerts an important feedback control not only on the reductase enzyme but also over the synthesis of LDL receptor. Thus when it is high, receptors are not synthesized and so uptake of more cholesterol from the plasma is blocked. This elaborate mechanism for regulating the cholesterol content of cells is necessary in view of the profound effect of the sterol on the fluidity of membranes and the limited storage facilities. Apart from its role in all cell membranes, cholesterol serves as precursor for the synthesis of bile acids in the liver and of steroid hormones in steroid-secreting endocrine glands.

Measurement of ^{125}I-labelled LDL bound to specific receptors on the membrane of mononuclear white cells has shown that heterozygotes for FH have only about half of the normal number of receptors. Not all genetic mutations of the gene coding for the receptor protein result in total inability to bind LDL; some may well produce only partially defective proteins. A further variant is known in which the receptor binds the LDL but fails to internalize the complex.

In addition to the specific receptor-operated cellular uptake, LDL is degraded also by a low affinity, non-saturable process which occurs at similar rates in normal and FH subjects. However, in the latter relatively more LDL is scavenged by macrophages which seems to predispose them to accumulation in xanthomas.

Treatment

The aim of therapy clearly must be to lower the serum cholesterol. Dietary treatment is wholly inadequate, since the most that can be achieved is a 10 per cent reduction. A bile acid sequestrant such as cholestyramine, given in fairly large doses over long periods, which binds bile acids within the intestinal lumen and prevents their reabsorption, has been reported in one study to lower the serum cholesterol by 20 per cent. The drain on cholesterol by faecal excretion of bile acids is believed to stimulate hepatic synthesis of LDL receptors in order to satisfy the organ's requirements for the sterol. Such an increase in receptors (which may not be under the control of the same gene as those in other tissues) would tend to lower the LDL cholesterol level in the plasma. The objective of current research is to combine bile acid sequestrant therapy with a drug capable of inhibiting cholesterol synthesis. Compactin, an analogue of mevalonic acid, inhibits the rate-limiting reductase and has shown promise in lowering the plasma cholesterol in experimental animals.

Additional Questions

1. How would you interpret a serum cholesterol of 8·8 mmol. ℓ^{-1} and

a serum triglyceride of 38 mmol. ℓ^{-1}?

2. Explain why the FH gene manifests a dominant inheritance. In what circumstances would the gene fail to be recognized as 'dominant'?

Further Reading

Havel, R. J., Goldstein, J. L. and Brown, M. S. (1980), Lipoprotein and lipid transport, *Metabolic Control and Disease*, eds Bondy, P. K. and Rosenberg, L. E. pp. 411–433, W. B. Saunders Co., Philadelphia.

Case 14

Case History

Janet P., aged 37, first consulted her doctor in 1972 because of 'indigestion', later diagnosed as duodenal ulcer. In September, 1974 she was seen at her home complaining of violent pain in her left flank and shortly afterwards she passed a stone. She was well until February, 1982 when she had another attack of renal colic, this time on the right. She was then referred to hospital for investigation.

Examination

The patient was of normal height and weight. She was not anaemic.

CVS	Pulse 76 per minute regular.
	Blood pressure 140/95 mmHg (lying).
	Heart sounds normal.
RS	Chest clear.
AS	No masses or tenderness.

X-ray of skull, chest, abdomen and long bones revealed no evidence of metabolic bone disease.

Laboratory Investigations

Investigation	Result	Reference range
March 1–5, 1982.		
Haemoglobin (g/dl)	14·5	13·0 – 17·0
White cells ($10^9 . \ell^{-1}$)	6·3	4·0 – 11·0
Differential count	normal	
Protein (g. ℓ^{-1})	65	62 – 82
Albumin (g. ℓ^{-1})	43	35 – 50
Serum calcium (mmol. ℓ^{-1})	2·62, 2·55, 2·58	2·25 – 2·65
Serum phosphate (mmol. ℓ^{-1})	0·89, 0·94, 0·89	0·8 – 1·6
Serum urea (mmol. ℓ^{-1})	7·7	2·5 – 7·5
Serum uric acid (mmol. ℓ^{-1})	0·3	0·12 – 0·48
Serum alkaline phosphatase (mU. ℓ^{-1})	47	30 – 110
Creatinine clearance (ml. min^{-1})	90	75 – 115
Urine sterile, normal volume and pH		
Calcium balance: on a diet containing		
0·8–1·0g Ca, average urine Ca over 4 days	5·0mmol/24h	2·5 – 7·5

Continued on next page

Laboratory Investigations contd

Investigation	Result	Reference range
Subsequent investigations, March 8–10, 1982.		
Total serum calcium (mmol. ℓ^{-1})	2·60	2·25 – 2·65
Ultrafilterable calcium (mmol. ℓ^{-1})	1·55, 1·49, 1·51	1·28 ± 0·05
Serum Phosphate (mmol. ℓ^{-1})	0·92	0·8 – 1·6
Total urinary hydroxyproline (mg/24h)	120	<50
Urinary cyclic AMP (mmol/dl GF)	9·5	3·19 ± 0·68

Questions

1. What is the differential diagnosis on March 5th, 1982?
2. What conclusions can you draw from the subsequent investigations?
3. Are there any further investigations you would request before treatment is begun and what is the treatment?

Leading Questions

1. (a) What is the nature of the most commonly found renal stones?
   (b) In the absence of an analysis of the stone, can any type of calculus be considered unlikely on the basis of the patient's history and serum biochemistry?
   (c) Which renal and prerenal circumstances predispose to the formation of calculi?
   (d) Is malignant disease a likely cause of the calculi?
   (e) What conclusions can be drawn from the normal X-ray examination?
2. (a) What significance do you attach to the ionised calcium in this patient?
   (b) Is the serum phosphorus compatible with your interpretation of the serum calcium?
   (c) How does the cyclic AMP help in understanding the patient's signs and symptoms?
   (d) What is the origin of urinary hydroxyproline and what conclusions can be drawn from its excessive excretion?
   (e) Is this conclusion warranted in the light of the normal alkaline phosphatase?
   (f) Are duodenal ulcer and hypertension chance findings in this patient?

3. (a) What is the definitive investigation in corroboration of the most likely diagnosis?
   (b) What treatment does it give rise to?

Discussion

An eight year history of renal colic and passage of a small stone, following on the diagnosis of duodenal ulcer, is the central abnormality in this case. Renal calculi most often (about 70 per cent) consist of calcium salts, of uric acid (10 per cent) or magnesium ammonium phosphate. They are formed as a result of increased absorption of calcium or its release from bone, of excessive ingestion of oxalate in the diet or synthesis of uric acid. Alkalinization of the tubular fluid by ammonia generated by bacteria in the urinary tract or undue concentration of the urine favour precipitation. Local circumstances in the kidney such as anatomical abnormalities leading to stasis and acidic or alkaline urine predispose to stone formation.

The stone passed by the patient could not be analyzed. It is, however, unlikely to have been a urate stone which is usually formed in an acidic urine; also, the serum urate is not raised and there are no clinical features suggestive of gout. Sterility of the urine precludes bacterial formation of ammonia and hence precipitation of a magnesium stone from an alkaline urine. A calcium oxalate or phosphate stone is thus much more probable.

A large proportion (80 per cent) of patients presenting with recurrent calcium stones have idiopathic hypercalciuria, a condition with a strong familial incidence, a preponderance in males and, by definition, associated with normocalcaemia. The disorder reflects, in most cases, excessive dietary absorption of calcium. In other cases tubular reabsorption is inherently defective and the urinary loss of calcium evokes secondary hyperparathyroidism which stimulates renal production of 1,25 dihydroxycholecalciferol and increases calcium absorption.

Hypervitaminosis D also can cause precipitation of calcium stones and careful questioning of the patient should establish the existence of any food fads or medications. Similarly, the milk alkali syndrome, now rarely seen, must be considered in view of the patient's duodenal ulcer. There are many other causes of urolithiasis, including bone metastases, sarcoidosis and renal tubular acidosis.

Hyperparathyroidism

In this patient the urinary excretion of calcium is not high and in the absence of evidence of dietary excess, the long history of renal calculi leads one to think of primary hyperparathyroidism (HP). This disease is usually but not necessarily associated with hyper-calcaemia. On three separate occasions the total serum calcium was well within normal limits and hence this and the other laboratory data obtained on March 1–5 contribute nothing positive to our understanding of the patient's problem. The only abnormality is a slightly elevated blood urea which raises the possibility of kidney damage due to episodic hypercalcaemia.

The long-standing nature of the disorder, together with the normal haematology and biochemistry, virtually rule out a host of malignant diseases with hypercalcaemia and calcium stones as sequelae. X-ray examination fails to show any evidence of osteitis fibrosa, one of the possible manifestations of HP.

Serum calcium and phosphate

In the light of this dirth of positive information more investigations are clearly called for and they are directed towards parathyroid function. Since serum calcium levels are subject to fluctuations and may be within normal limits for long periods only suddenly to rise and precipitate a hypercalcaemic crisis, repeated calcium determi-nations are indicated. It must be borne in mind that serum calcium consists of two main fractions – the physiologically important ionic calcium and the fraction bound to albumin, not subject to regulation. In the presence of hypoalbuminaemia the latter fraction can lower the total serum calcium and so mask a rise in ionic calcium. Although many established cases of HP with normocalcaemia have been reported, hypercalcaemia is still the single most common and reliable indicator of the disease. In this patient, determination of the ultrafilterable (ionised) calcium revealed a distinct hypercal-caemia. Here it should be noted that if conclusions are to be drawn from such slight deviations from the norm, adherence to an impec-cable laboratory technique and use of an appropriate reference range are of paramount importance. The latter is claimed to be age-dependent and different for males and females and must, in any case, be established in the same laboratory; the former includes attention to the manner of taking blood without stasis which signifi-cantly raises the serum calcium.

The serum phosphate is of limited value in the diagnosis of HP. Since parathyroid hormone (PTH) reduces the tubular reabsorption of phosphate, one would expect a serum level below the normal range and this is often found; however, idiopathic hypercalcaemia is also associated with hypophosphataemia. In 20 per cent of established cases of HP serum phosphate is normal and in the presence of renal insufficiency it can be raised. On the other hand, if kidney function is normal, a serum phosphate $> 1 \cdot 15$ mmol. ℓ^{-1} can be taken as strong evidence against this disease. In chronic renal disease hyperphosphataemia leads to hypocalcaemia and hence to secondary HP.

Parathyroid function

Theoretically the most definite test for HP is the determination of circulating PTH. Few laboratories are able to do this test in a manner which ensures that only biologically active hormone, rather than peptide fragments, are assayed by this radioimmunological technique. Such fragments may be particularly prominent in a patient with kidney disease as a consequence of primary HP as well as in other cases. An alternative is measurement of urinary cyclic AMP, the second messenger generated by PTH stimulation of renal receptors. Expressed in terms of glomerular filtrate, the cyclic AMP excretion of patients appears to be clearly separated from the normal range and unaffected by renal impairment. (Broadus *et al*, 1977) In this patient the cyclic AMP offers conclusive evidence for HP which accounts for the raised ionic calcium and the renal calculi.

Three categories of patients are recognized: those with bone disease (osteitis fibrosa), patients presenting with renal calculi composed of calcium phosphate or oxalate, and a third group presenting with neither of these. Radiological demonstration of bone disease is possible only in a small proportion of cases even in the first category and the diagnosis is therefore entirely dependent on the biochemical data, particularly serum calcium. It is usually higher in such patients compared to the stone formers, an observation which has been ascribed to the presence of a rapidly growing and very active tumour. Thus overt bone disease becomes manifest after a relatively short period of only 1–3 years, whereas kidney disease is associated with a slowly growing tumour of low activity which gives rise to a much longer period free or almost free of symptoms.

Notwithstanding this classification of HP, most if not all patients have excess bone resorption, irrespective of their clinical presentation, differing only in degree. The plasma calcium correlates with the extent of bone disease. Alkaline phosphatase has long served as an indicator of bone disease, although its serum concentration rises significantly only relatively late in the disease process. In some cases, such as the present patient, urinary hydroxyproline is more useful in indicating active bone resorption despite her clinical status.

Quite frequently duodenal ulcer is associated with HP, while hypertension may be a true complication, being present in more than 50 per cent of patients. Hyperuricaemia, usually without gout, is common too, while acute pancreatitis occurs in about 10 per cent of patients.

In the present circumstances the case for HP is very strong and no further tests are required before a definitive neck exploration and biopsy of all four parathyroid glands is undertaken. Removal of any tumour or hypertrophied gland is essential to prevent renal damage due to prolonged hypercalcaemia.

Calcium homeostasis depends on the interaction, both direct and permissive, of PTH and vitamin D, the main features of which are shown in the accompanying figure in a simplified form (*Figure 14.1*).

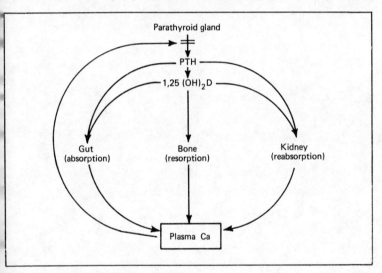

Figure 14.1 Regulation of plasma calcium

Additional Questions

1. Are there any hormones which may interfere with the interpretation of urinary cyclic AMP?
2. What are the most common symptoms of hypercalcaemia?

Further Reading

Alvioli, L. V. and Raisz, L. G. (1980) Hyperparathyroidism, in *Metabolic Control and Disease*, eds Bondy, P. K. and Rosenberg, L. E. 8th edn, pp. 1759–65, W. B. Saunders Co., Philadelphia.

Broadus, A. E., Mahaffey, J. E., Bartter, F. C. and Neer, R. M. (1977) Nephrogenous cyclic AMP as a parathyroid function test, *J. Clin. Invest.*, **60**, pp. 771–83.

Smith, L. H. (1978) Calcium-containing renal stones, *Kidney Int.*, **13**, pp. 383–89.

Case 15

Case History

Mr B. F., a 53-year-old widower, was admitted unconscious at midnight. He had been discovered by his son who reported that he had found an empty, open bottle of tablets and a bottle of whisky next to his father. Examination on admission was not helpful. Amongst other investigations the admitting casualty officer sent an urgent blood sample to the laboratory for blood glucose and alcohol which were reported to be 1·6 mmol. ℓ^{-1} and 32 mmol. ℓ^{-1} (160 mg/dl). The patient was therefore treated with an intravenous injection of 50 per cent glucose followed by a 5 per cent glucose infusion and he regained consciousness within a short time.

During the early morning the patient complained of being unwell and breathless.

Examination

The patient was visibly in some distress, tachypnoeic and obese.
CVS   Not anaemic or cyanosed. No oedema.
Pulse 88 per minute regular.
Blood pressure 130/80 mmHg (lying).
JVP not raised.
Heart sounds normal.
RS   Respiratory rate 30 per minute.
Chest clear.
AS and CNS Normal.

Laboratory Investigations

Results of investigations carried out 8 hours after admission.

Investigation	Result	Reference range
Plasma sodium (mmol. ℓ^{-1})	148	135–145
Plasma potassium (mmol. ℓ^{-1})	5·4	3·3–5·3
Plasma chloride (mmol. ℓ^{-1})	98	98–108
Plasma urea (mmol. ℓ^{-1})	5·1	2·5–7·5
Blood glucose (mmol. ℓ^{-1}) (random)	7·6	3·5–10
Arterial pH	7·12	7·36–7·44

Continued on next page

Laboratory Investigations contd

Arterial PO_2 (mm Hg)	95	80–105
Arterial PCO_2 (mm Hg)	18	35–47
Base excess	−23	±3
Plasma bicarbonate (mmol. ℓ^{-1})	6·0	22–30

Note: to convert PO_2, PCO_2 and the respective reference ranges to kPa divide by 7·5.

Questions

1. What was the differential diagnosis when the patient was first seen in casualty?
2. Why is the patient tachypnoeic?
3. What is the significance of the biochemical abnormalities found on the morning after admission?
4. What additional investigations would prove useful?
5. What treatment would you give?

Leading Questions

1. (a) What are the chief causes of unconsciousness?
   (b) Can any of these be eliminated by clinical examination? Is alcohol implicated? Which cause is the most likely in this patient?
   (c) What investigations could help to eliminate other causes?
   (d) What tests should be performed to confirm and further elucidate the likely diagnosis?
   (e) What are the main causes of hypoglycaemia?
2. (a) What are the causes of tachypnoea?
   (b) Which of these are likely to be found in a patient in or recovering from coma?
   (c) Do the blood gases indicate the nature of the respiratory disturbance?
3. (a) What is the nature of the acid base disturbance?
   (b) Why is the finding of normal plasma urea and blood glucose helpful in assessing the cause of the acid-base disturbance?
   (c) Is this a simple disturbance or has it been modified by homeostatic mechanisms?
   (d) What would you expect to be the effect of the various causes of tachypnoea on the arterial blood gas measurements? What cause best fits the results found in the patient?

   (e) Is the raised plasma sodium explicable in terms of another
        biochemical abnormality?
4. (a) What are the likely causes of the acid base abnormality
        found in this patient?
   (b) Do any of the biochemical results confirm or eliminate any of
        these causes?
   (c) Explain the meaning of negative base excess. What conclu-
        sions can be drawn from it?
   (e) Does the negative base excess suggest an important investi-
        gation which must be carried out?
   (f) What action would you take in respect of the tablets
        swallowed by this patient?
5. (a) What are the prime objectives of treating this condition?
   (b) What specific therapy is available to effect these objectives?
   (c) Are there are dangers or unwanted side effects of therapy?
   (d) What is the prognosis?

Discussion

When first seen in casualty the differential diagnosis is that of uncon-sciousness, causes of which include trauma, post-ictal states, cerebrovascular accidents, intracranial tumour, meningitis and encephalitis, diabetic ketoacidosis, non-ketotic hyperosmolar coma, hypoglycaemia, renal failure, hepatic failure, adrenal disease, alcohol intoxication and other poisoning. The finding of the empty bottle of tablets suggests that drug overdose should head the list in this patient. Drugs to be considered include salicylates, paracetamol, barbiturates and other hypnotics, tricyclic anti-depressants and benzodiazepines. In attempted suicide drugs are taken either singly or in combination and are frequently taken together with alcohol. With the lack of additional history or clinical evidence indicating a specific diagnosis a wide range of investiga-tions can be justified. The most urgent include blood count and white cell differential to exclude infection, X-ray of the skull to exclude trauma or its sequelae, urea and electrolytes, blood sugar, serum salicylate and paracetamol and blood alcohol. A lumbar puncture should be performed if papilloedema is absent. Urine should be examined for sugar and ketones and a sample of the first urine obtained should be kept for drug screening: drugs and their metabolites are nearly always more concentrated in urine. Liver function tests may be required if all the above investigations are negative and can serve as a useful baseline for possible later manifestations of paracetamol poisoning.

The causes of hypoglycaemia

The finding of hypoglycaemia and the rapid clinical response to intravenous glucose lead one to consider the causes of hypo-glycaemia. In the age group of the patient the differential diagnosis would include insulinoma and deliberate or accidental insulin over-dose, drugs and alcohol, hypopituitarism, adrenal insufficiency and reactive hypoglycaemia in diabetes or postgastrectomy. A number of drugs can cause hypoglycaemia, the most obvious of which are the oral hypoglycaemic agents; the sulphonylureas (chlor-propamide, tolbutamide etc.) and the biguanides (phenformin and metformin). Other drugs include salicylates. The probability that the hypoglycaemia in the patient was at least in part drug induced was in fact strengthened when the tablets originally in bottle turned out to be phenformin. The role of ethanol in this patient is complex for

besides causing hypoglycaemia in its own right, ethanol can poten-
tiate the hypoglycaemic action of other drugs.

Nature of the respiratory disturbance

The onset of breathlessness and feeling unwell could be due to the
ingestion of certain drugs, aspiration pneumonia secondary to
coma, cardiac failure and pulmonary oedema or to psychiatric
causes, in particular anxiety. Cardiac failure, aspiration pneumonia
and other chest pathology can be excluded by physical and
radiological examination. Anxiety is a likely cause in a patient who
has made a failed attempt at suicide. However, the arterial blood
gas analysis reveals that the patient has an acute metabolic acidosis
with a decrease in pH, plasma bicarbonate and base excess,
whereas in acute hyperventilation from anxiety a respiratory
alkalosis would be found with increased pH, decreased P_{CO_2} and
normal base excess. The bicarbonate is low because in buffering
the increased hydrogen ion it forms carbonic acid which in turn
decomposes to CO_2 and water: at the same time the acid which is
responsible for the metabolic acidosis replaces the bicarbonate as
the counterion to plasma sodium. The negative base excess
increases correspondingly. A separate effect of the acidaemia is
stimulation of the respiratory centre: the resulting hyperventilation
rapidly removes CO_2 and in 6–12 hours compensates, at least
partially, for the fall in pH that the fixed acid would otherwise have
produced. In rare cases of metabolic acidosis hyperventilation can
be so pronounced as to reduce the P_{CO_2} to less than 10 mmHg
(1·3kPa).

Metabolic acidosis

Metabolic acidosis is caused by a primary accumulation of non-
volatile acid, loss of base or by a combination of the two. Accumulation of acid can arise from increased production, e.g., β-hydroxy-
butyrate and acetoacetate in diabetic ketoacidosis and starvation or
of lactic acid in shock, hypoxia, ingestion of various drugs and
several inborn errors of carbohydrate metabolism. Decreased
excretion of acid by the kidneys in chronic renal failure or renal
tubular acidosis will also cause an accumulation of acid. Loss of base
(bicarbonate) occurs principally in gastrointestinal disorders
associated with severe chronic diarrhoea or fistulae.

Examination of the biochemical findings in the patient will eliminate several of the causes of metabolic acidosis. The presentation with hypoglycaemia and the normal blood sugar found in the second sample taken 8 hours after admission when the patient was acidotic eliminates completely any possibility of diabetic ketacidosis. The normal urea would eliminate chronic renal failure. However, a greatly raised anion gap $[(Na+K)-(Cl+HCO_3)]$ (48·7 mmol. ℓ^{-1}, normal 10–18 mmol. ℓ^{-1}) signifies the presence of other unmeasured anions. In these circumstances the most likely 'missing' anion is lactate which should therefore be measured in the patient.

Lactic acidosis

Quantitative definitions of lactic acidosis are arbitrary and values given by different authors vary. Cohen and Woods (*see* further reading) divide lactic acidosis clinically into two types, A and B. Type A is associated with and the result of tissue hypoxia due either to poor perfusion or to low PO_2 of the arterial blood. All other causes of lactic acidosis, including a subgroup caused by the ingestion of drugs or toxic agents, constitute Type B. Ethanol is especially relevant as the patient's blood level was high. Apart from generating acetic acid in the course of its oxidation, alcohol reduces NAD to NADH with consequent widespread metabolic derangements, including a partial inhibition of the citric acid cycle and excessive formation of lactate. Salicylate poisoning may be associated with excess of lactic acid and the hypoglycaemic agents phenformin and metformin, especially the former, are well known to produce a severe lactic acidosis. This was the case in this patient who had been prescribed phenformin for his Type II non-insulin dependent diabetes. Ethanol and phenformin act synergistically in raising blood lactate and phenformin treated diabetics have a reduced ethanol tolerance.

The precise pathogenesis of both types of lactic acidosis is still unclear. In Type A hypoxia will lead to increased anaerobic glycolysis particularly in muscle and hence accumulation of pyruvate and lactate. There is considerable evidence that a decrease in lactate removal by the liver either by oxidation or gluconeogenesis is also important. The pathogenesis of Type B acidosis is variable depending on the aetiology. The metabolic effects of phenformin by which it produces lactic acidosis are not understood but it does not appear to act by inhibiting tissue oxidation. There is some evidence that phenformin reduces lactate uptake by the liver and also gluconeogenesis possibly by independent mechanisms.

Treatment

Correction of metabolic acidosis is not simple. In some cases such as diabetic ketoacidosis, treatment of the primary condition will lead to the removal of the excess hydrogen ion by metabolism and specific treatment of the acidosis is not required unless it is so severe as to be life-threatening. However, alkali therapy is potentially dangerous as it may result in metabolic alkalosis in these cases. In Type A lactic acidosis, therapeutic emphasis is placed on improving tissue oxygenation and combating shock as well as the acidosis. Treatment of Type B lactic acidosis is with bicarbonate given as an infusion to restore the pH to normality in 2–6 hours and then to maintain it. Haemodialysis may be required. Normalization of the pH may have unwanted side effects which include a shift of the oxyhaemoglobin dissociation curve to the left thus reducing tissue oxygenation and increasing the rate of glycolysis and lactate production. It is not surprising therefore that the value and method of alkalinization of patients with lactic acidosis is still questioned and the mortality of Type B is as high as 80 per cent.

Additional Questions

1. What are the normal pathways for the production and removal of lactate? How are they controlled?
2. What are the important biochemical investigations which should be carried out on a suspected case of drug overdose?

Further Reading

Cohen, R. D. and Woods, H. F. (1976). *Clinical and Biochemical Aspects of Lactic Acidosis*, pp. 40–76, Blackwell Scientific Publications, Oxford.

Case 16

Case History

A 39-year-old man who worked in his own car breakers yard first presented to his general practitioner with generalized abdominal pain which was treated symptomatically. Several months later he returned and on this occasion he complained of several symptoms, including headache, insomnia and depression. He was referred to a psychiatrist who elicited the additional history of difficulty in concentration when doing the paperwork associated with his business and of forgetting essential information.

The abdominal pain did not respond to treatment and the patient developed some muscle pain and generalized weakness. An episode of very severe colic and vomiting resulted in an admission to hospital.

Examination

The patient was pale with definite clinical anaemia. He responded to questions slowly and showed some signs of disorientation.

CVS   Pulse 60 per minute regular.
          Blood pressure 140/90 mmHg (lying).
          Heart sounds normal.
CNS   Mild peripheral muscular weakness.
          No sensory abnormalities.

Laboratory Investigations

Investigation	Result	Reference range
Plasma sodium (mmol. ℓ^{-1})	143	134 – 145
Plasma potassium (mmol. ℓ^{-1})	4·2	3·3–5·3
Plasma chloride (mmol. ℓ^{-1})	104	98 – 108
Plasma urea (mmol. ℓ^{-1})	9·3	2·5 – 7·5
Urine protein (by dipstick)	+ +	negative
Urine glucose (by dipstick)	+	negative
Haemoglobin (g.dl^{-1})	9·5	13 – 17
RBC ($\times 10^{12}$. ℓ^{-1})	3·0	4·5 – 6·5
MCV (fl)	68	80 – 92
MCHC (%)	30	31 – 35
PCV (1. ℓ^{-1})	0·32	0·40 – 0·49

Questions

1. What is the differential diagnosis?
2. What further tests should be carried out to distinguish the various possible causes?
3. What treatment would you prescribe and what is the prognosis?

Leading Questions

1. (a) What signs and symptoms would indicate that this patient is suffering from an organic rather than a functional psychosis?
   (b) What causes of organic psychoses should be considered in this patient?
   (c) Which signs and symptoms indicate a specific organic disorder in this patient?
2. (a) Which biochemical pathway is most likely to be affected in this patient given the available evidence?
   (b) How is it controlled?
   (c) Which steps in this pathway are inhibited in the patient and what are the biochemical consequences?
   (d) What other diseases manifest interference of the same pathway?
   (e) What are the characteristic biochemical findings in these diseases?
   (f) Explain how the block of the synthetic pathway leads to the haematological manifestations.
   (g) What would you expect to see in the blood film?
3. (a) In what circumstances is active treatment indicated?
   (b) What do you consider to be the first step which should be taken in treatment?
   (c) What is the aim of active treatment and how is it achieved?
   (d) Are there any potential hazards?
   (e) How would you monitor the therapy?
   (f) Does the patient's age affect the prognosis?

Discussion

The presentation of the patient with mixed psychiatric and physical symptoms suggests that the first stage in the diagnosis is to distinguish whether he has a 'functional' or an 'organic' cause for his neuropsychiatric signs and symptoms. In this case the combination of impairment of intellectual ability with poor memory, inability to concentrate, mild disorientation and headache is strongly indicative of an organic cause for his illness. Diseases which should be considered include encephalitis, tuberculous meningitis, uraemia, hypertensive encephalopathy, metabolic and toxic causes. The symptoms of severe colic, vomiting and generalized weakness would suggest a toxic cause and the patient's anaemia and his occupation would make lead poisoning the probable diagnosis. The hepatic porphyrias should be considered as an alternative possibility since psychiatric disturbances are relatively common in patients with acute intermittent porphyria and hereditary coproporphyria. These patients have other signs and symptoms similar to those found in lead poisoning, including abdominal pain, constipation, vomiting and peripheral motor neuropathy.

Haem synthesis

In order to differentiate between lead poisoning annd porphyria it is necessary to understand haem synthesis (*Figure 16.1*) and the effects of lead on the various steps in the pathway. The first step is the formation of δ-aminolaevulinic acid (ALA) from succinylCoA and glycine catalyzed by the enzyme ALA synthetase. Two molecules of ALA are then joined to form porphobilinogen (PBG) by the enzyme ALA dehydratase, an enzyme which is highly sensitive to lead. Four molecules of PBG are coupled to form uroporphyrinogen III which in turn is metabolized to coproporhyrinogen III. In the final stages of haem synthesis the coproporphyrinogen is converted first to protoporphyrin IX and then to haem with the incorporation of iron by the enzyme ferrochelatase. This latter enzyme is also highly sensitive to lead. The control of haem synthesis is complex but a major role is played by feedback inhibition of ALA synthetase by haem.

Accumulation of intermediates

The biochemical consequences of lead poisoning can be predicted from the above description. ALA accumulates in all tissues as a result of a combination of the removal of the haem feedback control

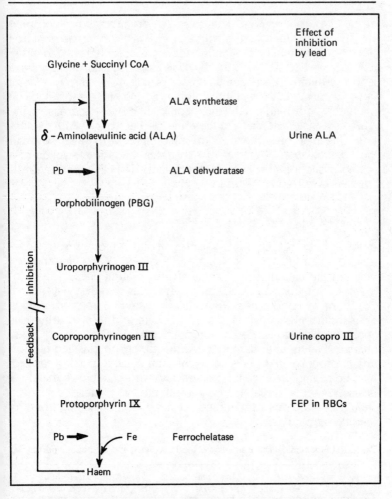

Figure 16.1 Pathway of synthesis of haem showing enzymes affected in lead poisoning and the biochemical effects

of ALA synthetase and the inhibition by lead of ALA dehydratase and is excreted in large quantities in the urine. The major sources of ALA in the urine are liver and bone marrow. The inhibition of ALA dehydratase is one of the earliest demonstrable effects of lead occurring at blood lead levels of <1.0 μmol. ℓ^{-1} (<20 μg/dl). A second effect is the accumulation of protoporphyrin in the erythrocytes. It is present as the zinc complex *in vivo* and can be measured by extraction and fluorimetry or more directly by microscale fluorimetry of the red cells. On extraction the zinc is lost and the red cell protoporphyrin is referred to as free erythrocyte protoporphyrin (FEP). It is important to note that FEP is also increased in iron deficiency anaemia although it does not reach the levels found in lead poisoning: FEP > 100 μg/dl whole blood is usually indicative of lead poisoning. The accumulation of protoporphyrin may seem a little surprising in view of the inhibition of one of the early steps on the pathway by lead but the inhibition is lifted by the increase in the ALA pool which stems from the enhanced activity of ALA synthetase. One final consequence of the inhibition of ferrochelatase is that the accumulation of precursor substrates leads to activation of a normally silent pathway and the production of coproporphyrin III which is excreted in the urine.

Urinary porphyrias in other diseases

In the hepatic porphyrias the excretion of haem precursors varies according to the type of disorder (*Table 16.1*) and depends on whether the patient is in an acute attack or latent phase. Measurements of urinary ALA, PBG and porphyrins together with faecal porphyrin are performed. PBG must be tested on fresh urine since on standing it is converted to porphobilin and in acid urine it is spontaneously converted to uroporphyrin. PBG is raised in all attacks of acute intermittent and variegate porphyrias and hereditary coproporphyria but is not significantly raised in many cases of lead poisoning. In acute intermittent and variegate porphyrias PBG is also raised in the latent phase. With the aid of these tests there should be little difficulty in differentiating lead poisoning from the hepatic porphyrias.

Table 16.1 Biochemical Differentiation of lead poisoning and the hepatic porphyrias

	Lead Poisoning	Acute intermittent porphyria	Variegate porphyria	Hereditary coproporphyria
Urine PBG	±	++(±)	++(±)	+(±)
Urine ALA	++	++(±)	++(±)	+(−)
Urine porphyrin	++	+(−)	++(±)	+(−)
Faecal porphyrin	−	±(−)	+(±)	+(+)
Erythrocyte protoporphyrin (FEP)	++	−(−)	−(−)	−(−)

Screening tests. Symbols in brackets indicate findings in latent disease.

Porphyrins may be excreted in the urine in several other diseases. These causes of porphyrinuria include the erythropoietic porphyrias, certain liver diseases, e.g., infectious hepatitis, cirrhosis and haemochromatosis, acute and chronic alcoholism, haemolytic, aplastic and pernicious anaemias and poisoning with various chemical agents. In none of these is there any excretion of either ALA or PBG.

Body lead

These indirect tests of the effects of lead poisoning remain important although it is possible to measure lead directly in blood. At least 90 per cent of the lead in blood is bound to the red cell; lead is therefore measured in whole blood and not in serum or plasma. There is rather poor correlation between the blood lead and the clinical state of the patient as the lead concentration reflects recent exposure rather than overall body burden which is mainly in the bone. Lead is difficult to measure and the assay is usually performed in specialised laboratories. Contamination from external lead sources is always a problem, particularly if samples are taken by skin puncture.

Though lead is widely distributed in the body there are few biochemical abnormalities observed, even in severe poisoning, other than the effects on the haem pathway. In children and less frequently in adults, renal tubular damage can cause a Fanconi syndrome with glucosuria, amino aciduria and phosphaturia often with proteinuria. Chronic renal failure is rare and the raised plasma urea in this patient is most likely to be from mild dehydration associated with vomiting.

There are a number of haematological findings in chronic lead poisoning the most common, but not invariable, being anaemia which is usually microcytic hypochromic. Serum iron and TIBC are usually normal. Classically basophilic stippling of erythrocytes is seen in the blood film but this is absent in 40 per cent of patients even with high blood lead levels; there is no correlation between the extent of stippling and the blood lead concentration. Basophilic stippling, which is due to unresorbed polysomes and their associated RNA, is not specific and can be found in other haematological disorders. Red cell life is shortened and a mild reticulocytosis is usually present.

Therapy

Treatment depends on the patient's clinical condition but it is essential to identify the source of lead and to remove the patient from it. If the blood level is very high, $>5.8\,\mu$mol. ℓ^{-1}., ($>120\,\mu$g/ml) in an adult or $>4.0\,\mu$mol. ℓ^{-1}., ($>83\,\mu$g/ml) in children, treatment with chelating agents should be tried. EDTA is normally given intravenously at doses of 50–75 mg/kg body weight/24 hours in a saline drip followed by oral treatment with edethamil calcium disodium 2 g b.d. Alternative chelating agents include penicillamine and dimercaprol. Problems with chelation therapy include renal damage and trace metal deficiency. As the greater part of lead is sequestered in the bone and is inaccessible to chelating agents only a relatively small pool of lead is easily removed. Thus repeated courses of chelation therapy may be necessary and it may take several years for the body lead to fall to acceptable levels.

Symptomatic treatment may be required. Abdominal colic is relieved by the administration of calcium gluconate. The use of drugs such as barbiturates must be avoided until the diagnosis is firmly established as they could cause a worsening of the clinical condition if the patient had one of the forms of hepatic porphyria.

Treatment may be monitored by the use of any of the diagnostic tests. Blood lead, urinary ALA and coproporphyrin fall rapidly during chelation therapy but rise gradually when treatment stops. FEP on the other hand falls much more slowly, reflecting red cell turnover. FEP is probably the best and simplest means of assessing the reduction in body lead and may take years to return to normal levels. This reflects the slow continuous release of lead from bone consequent on remodelling.

The prognosis in an adult patient with lead poisoning is good given effective therapy; even the peripheral neuropathy will be cured. In children, on the other hand, lead poisoning is often followed by neurological sequelae including mental retardation. The maximum permissible levels of lead in children remain controversial.

Additional Questions

1. What is the interrelationship between lead and iron metabolism?
2. What are the functions of haem outside the bone marrow?
3. Why are porphyrins excreted in some liver diseases?

Further Reading

Hamilton, A., Hardy, H. L. and Finkel, A. J. (1983) *Industrial Toxicology*, 2nd edn revised, pp. 62–87 John Wright, Boston.

Case 17

Case History

Robert A. was admitted to a children's hospital at 20 days of age. He had been born at term after a normal pregnancy, birth weight 3550g, and developed normally on a cow's milk preparation until day 15 when he vomited several times. Subsequently he had become apathetic, refused his feeds, vomited and had some loose stools. Vomiting was unconnected with his feeds and was not projectile.

On admission his weight was 3100g. He was clinically dehydrated and there was a greyish cyanosis of his lips. A weak pulse and cold perspiration indicated peripheral vascular failure. Blood was taken for determination of electrolytes and he was given an intravenous drip of isotonic glucose saline. Vomiting and diarrhoea ceased within a few hours of rehydration. Abdominal palpation revealed no tumour.

Three days later he was discharged with a diagnosis of gastro-enteritis, having begun to put on weight. He was progressing satisfactorily until at age 2½ months he developed a mild bronchial infection. He started vomiting and two days later he had to be readmitted in a state of collapse. After collecting blood for electrolyte determination, rehydration was commenced and he was treated with antibiotics. The first sample of urine passed was collected for analysis of electrolytes.

Laboratory investigations

Investigation	Day of first admission	second admission	Reference range
Blood glucose (mmol. ℓ^{-1}) (fasting)	4·5	—	2·5 – 5·0
Serum sodium (mmol. ℓ^{-1})	114	128	135 – 145
Serum potassium (mmol. ℓ^{-1})	6·9	6·0	4·0 – 5·6
Serum chloride (mmol. ℓ^{-1})	96	—	95 – 105
Serum urea (mmol. ℓ^{-1})	13·5	15·2	2·5 – 7·5
Urine sodium (mmol. ℓ^{-1})	—	110	*
Urine potassium (mmol. ℓ^{-1})	—	5·9	*

* Urine sodium and potassium output depend on intake, which is unknown in this case. Urinary excretion of these ions must be evaluated with reference to serum concentrations.

Questions

1. What is the differential diagnosis?
2. What further tests would aid the diagnosis?
3. Is there a specific therapy you would institute? What are the potential dangers and how can they be avoided?
4. What is the aetiology and pathogenesis of the condition?
5. How is treatment controlled in the long term?

Leading Questions

1. (a) What are the more common causes of vomiting and diarrhoea in infants?
   (b) The vomiting is not projectile and is unconnected with the feeds, it is not associated with constipation; there is no palpable abdominal mass: what conclusions can be drawn from this?
   (c) If the degree of dehydration seemed excessive in relation to the vomiting and diarrhoea, what other factors should be considered?
   (d) Can any conclusion be drawn from the cessation of vomiting and diarrhoea within a few hours of rehydration?
   (e) How do you account for the collapse at $2\frac{1}{2}$ months?
   (f) Which is the outstanding abnormality in the laboratory investigations? What are its likely causes in the light of the patient's age? Which physiological mechanism is likely to be implicated?
2. (a) Is there any evidence of renal failure?
   (b) What specific investigations are available for assessing alternative causes of disturbed sodium homeostasis?
3. (a) The immediate need is clearly to replace the fluid loss. What additional measures are indicated?
   (b) What is the danger implicit in the therapy? Could daily clinical and/or biochemical assessment lessen it?
   (c) What is the long-term treatment?
4. (a) What substances are normally produced by the organ implicated in the condition?
   (b) What are their biological effects or functions?
   (c) How does their biosynthesis relate them to each other?
   (d) How is their output controlled?
   (e) What tentative conclusions can be drawn from the illness beginning in the neonatal period?

(f) Would a metabolic block somewhere in the synthetic pathway account for the clinical and biochemical observations?

(g) Do you know of any other clinical manifestations sometimes seen in this condition?

Discussion

An infant, seemingly healthy at birth and gaining weight in the first 2 weeks of postnatal life, starts vomiting on day 15. Thereafter he loses interest in his feeds, has vomiting and diarrhoea, and becomes dehydrated. He has lost more than 10 per cent of his birth weight. At this stage, gastroenteritis, pyloric stenosis, a metabolic abnormality and adrenocortical malfunction must be considered. Poor appetite, the nature of the vomiting, absence of constipation and no palpable abdominal mass render pyloric stenosis unlikely. The plasma urea on the day of first admission confirm the clinical evidence of dehydration. Following rehydration on his first admission he seems well (hence a metabolic defect is less likely), but a mild infection precipitates another episode of dehydration which brings him back to hospital in a state of collapse. This course of events is much more suggestive of adrenocortical insufficiency. On second admission the patient's hyponatraemia can be seen to be concurrent with an inappropriate urinary excretion of sodium – a strong indication of a failure of aldosterone-mediated electrolyte regulation or of renal disease. Transient hypoaldosteronism, possibly due to delayed enzyme formation, a renal tubular insensitivity to the hormone or Addison's disease, extremely rare in infants and children, should be considered, but the most likely cause of the symptoms is congenital adrenal hyperplasia (CAH).

Steroid assay

In the diagnosis of CAH the availability of specific steroid analyses has almost entirely replaced the need for measurements in urine of pregnanetriol, 17-oxosteroids or the 11-oxygenation index. The most useful plasma steroids for CAH diagnosis are 17-α-hydroxyprogesterone (17OHP) and 11-deoxycortisol (11-DC), which are elevated in the 21-hydroxylase and 11-hydroxylase deficiencies respectively. These two assays will diagnose more than 98 per cent of all cases of CAH. It is also useful to measure cortisol in these patients, since in other causes of adrenal insufficiency in infancy 17OHP, 11-DC and cortisol will all be low. 17OHP can be raised to similar values as those found in CAH in sick premature infants and is not specific in these cases. ACTH assay, when available, will confirm the absence of feedback control by cortisol when ACTH is high and establish the reason for the overproduction of cortisol precursors and adrenal androgens.

Treatment

There is an urgent need to rehydrate the patient with IV saline and to treat the precipitating cause, usually infection. Apart from this, there is an immediate and longterm requirement to replace the absent glucocorticoid and mineralocorticoid where necessary. The former is usually achieved with cortisol, both to suppress ACTH secretion and prevent synthesis of excess adrenal androgens, and ensure the necessary peripheral hormone action. Undertreatment will lead to rapidly advancing bone age, premature fusion of the epiphyses and signs and symptoms of chronic Addison's disease; overtreatment, on the other hand, leads to iatrogenic Cushing's syndrome. Therapy can be monitored by multiple determinations of 170HP in plasma or saliva, there being a direct correlation between the two and saliva being a highly suitable sample in children. Several specimens should be taken throughout the day to allow for circadian variation in the ACTH output.

A mineralocorticoid will be required in the acute phase in all patients but only a proportion of salt losers will require continuation of this therapy when adequate glucocorticoid replacement has been achieved. Measurement of plasma electrolytes is too insensitive to establish the adequacy of replacement and optimum therapy is ensured by renin determination made during periods of controlled sodium balance. If a patient requires mineralocorticoid, this, like cortisol, is needed for life.

Genetic linkage of the 21-hydroxylase gene and the HLA-B determinant on the sixth chromosome has been established. This has allowed the identification of heterozygotes in affected families and of undiagnosed cases. Antenatal diagnosis is also now possible, both by HLA typing and measurement of steroids in amniotic fluid. No evidence for linkage with HLA types has been found for other forms of CAH.

Steroid synthesis

The adrenal cortex produces glucocorticoids, progesterone, aldosterone, androgens and oestrogens. All derive from cholesterol by successive oxidation and hydroxylation, the availability of cholesterol for these reactions being controlled by ACTH. Two oxidative reactions (A, B) yield progesterone (*Figure 17.1*). Thereafter, specific hydroxylations (C-F) introduce OH groups at carbons 17, 21, 11 and 18, producing a variety of intermediates and ultimately

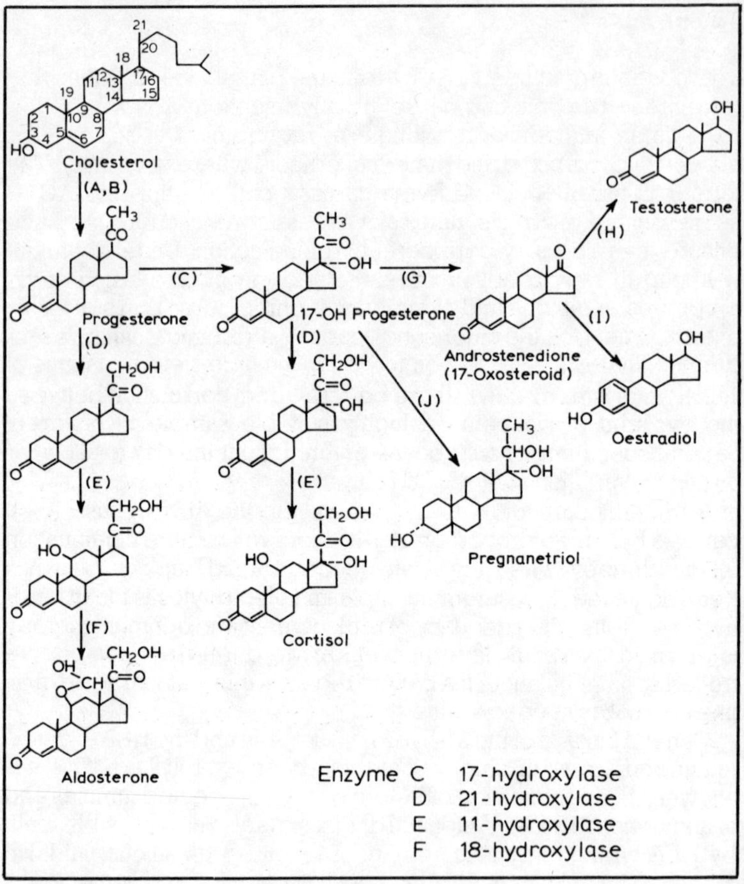

Figure 17.1 Steroid synthesis in the adrenal cortex

cortisol and aldosterone. A subsidiary pathway leads from 17-hydroxyprogesterone by an oxidative removal of C_{20} and C_{21} (reaction G) to androgens and oestrogens.

To understand the pathophysiology of CAH it is helpful to remember that the 11-OH group confers glucocorticoid activity on the steroid, while the 11-deoxy compounds tend to be mineralocorticoids. In aldosterone itself the 11-OH has, of course, given rise to an oxygen-based 5-membered ring involving C_{18}. Hydroxylation at C_{17} does not alter the biological function but is an essential step in the synthesis of both cortisol and androgens.

An inadequate production of cortisol and the consequent failure of feedback control of ACTH release by the pituitary leads to excessive mobilization of cholesterol and hyperplasia of the adrenocortical tissue in an attempt to step up the synthesis of the glucocorticoid. Oxidations and hydroxylations proceed at an accelerated pace up to a metabolic block created by a defective or absent hydroxylase. If the block is incomplete, some cortisol will be synthesized and eventually the ACTH release brought under control. If the hydroxylase is totally inactive, ACTH stimulation will go unchecked. In any event, intermediates proximal to the block will build up either in the cortex or in extracortical tissue and so open up metabolic pathways which are normally insignificant. We can see from *Figure 17.1* that a defective 17, 21 or 11-hydroxylase will have this effect. Of these three enzymes the 21-hydroxylase is most frequently implicated. The concentration of 17-OH progesterone will rise until it compensates for the low affinity which enzymes G and J can be assumed to have for this substrate and the respective reactions will produce the increased amounts of 17-oxosteroids and pregnanetriol found in the urine.

Excessive production of androgens leads to virilization which is especially prominent in female infants but is often missed in males in the first few weeks of life. The latter are, therefore, more liable to die in an Addisonian crisis before the diagnosis has been made and salt balance restored. Another possible consequence of an unchecked anterior pituitary activity is over-production of MSH and hence pigmentation of the skin.

Salt balance

Involvement of aldosterone in the pathology of CAH is more difficult to understand. In the first place, aldosterone output is regulated by the kidney via renin/angiotensin and directly by the plasma Na and K concentration rather than by ACTH. While aldosterone cannot be synthesized in the complete absence of either the 21 or the 11 (or indeed the 18) hydroxylase, the small quantities required to maintain normal salt balance might well be produced by a partially defective enzyme. This is the case in some patients; yet others present in an Addisonian crisis, but once this has been overcome and ACTH output returned to normal levels, such patients may remain in apparent Na and K balance for long periods. Two possible explanations have been offered for the temporary salt loss. According to one, certain steroids with a mild anti-aldosterone activity, e.g., progesterone, produced in excess under the intense stimulation by ACTH, overwhelm the small but usually adequate amounts of aldosterone. The other hypothesis invokes the production of a natriuretic steroid which also stops when ACTH output is curbed.

Additional Questions

1. In what respects, if any, would the biochemical and clinical manifestations of a deficiency of 11-hydroxylase differ from those of 21-hydroxylase?
2. How would you establish that enlargement of the phallus and hirsutism in a male infant is due to CAH rather than a testicular tumour?

Further Reading

Brook, C. G. D. (1981) Congenital adrenal hyperplasia, *Clinical Paediatric Endocrinology*, ed. Brook, C. G. D., pp. 453–464, Blackwell Scientific Publications, Oxford.

Case 18

Case History

Mr C. L. was first admitted to hospital at the age of 46 complaining of muscle cramps, weakness, vertigo, nausea and vomiting. In the past he had been noticed to have a trace of proteinuria at a pre-employment medical but this had not been followed up at that time. Questioning revealed that the patient drank between 15 and 20 cups of beverages a day, had nocturia 2–3 times nightly for 3 years and had been passing increased amounts of urine. He had also been falling asleep after returning home from work. The patient commented that he had been adding increased quantities of salt to his food.

Examination

The patient was clinically anaemic and had a markedly dry skin with reduced skin turgor.
CVS   Pulse 82 per minute regular.
        Blood pressure 130/80 mmHg (lying).
        Heart sounds normal.
No other significant clinical findings.
Biochemical and haematological investigations at this time are shown below.

Progress

Treatment was commenced with intravenous saline and the patient placed on a low protein diet. Over the next few years there were several further similar admissions. Results of biochemical investigations on a subsequent admission aged 49 are also shown below.

Laboratory investigations

Investigation	Results Age 46	Age 49	Reference Range
Plasma sodium (mmol. ℓ^{-1})	128	120	135 – 145
Plasma potassium (mmol. ℓ^{-1})	4·6	4·2	3·3 – 5·3
Plasma chloride (mmol. ℓ^{-1})	88	81	98 – 108
Plasma bicarbonate (mmol. ℓ^{-1})	18	16	22 – 30

Continued on next page

130

Laboratory Investigations contd

Investigation	Result		Reference range
Plasma urea (mmol. ℓ^{-1})	66	54	2·5 – 7·5
Plasma osmolality (mmol. kg^{-1})	314	285	280 – 295
Serum protein (g. ℓ^{-1})	68	64	62 – 82
Serum albumin (g. ℓ^{-1})	40	38	37 – 47
Serum globulin (g. ℓ^{-1})	28	26	20 – 37
Serum calcium (mmol. ℓ.)	2·2	2·3	2·25 – 2·65
Serum phosphate (mmol. ℓ.)	1·9	2·2	1·1 – 1·8
Serum creatinine (μmol. ℓ^{-1})	920	1120	45 – 125
Serum urate (mmol. ℓ^{-1})	0·56		0·18 – 0·48
Blood glucose (mmol. ℓ^{-1}) (random)	5·2		3·5 – 10
Urine osmolality (mmol. kg^{-1})	320	295	500 – 800[a]
Urine protein (by dipstick)	+ +	+ +	negative
Urine sodium (mmol. 24h^{-1})	127	160	80 – 225[a]
Urine volume (ml. 24h^{-1})	3500	3150	1000 – 1500[b]
Urine glucose (by dipstick)	negative		negative
Creatinine clearance (ml.min^{-1}.1·73 m^{-2})	7·3	5·5	85 – 150
Haemoglobin (g. dl^{-1})	10·8	8·5	13 – 17
RBC (10^{12}. ℓ^{-1})	3·72	3·1	4·5 – 6·5
MCHC (g. dl)	33	31	31 – 45
MCH (pg)	29	27·5	27 – 32

[a] On normal diet.
[b] On normal fluid intake. Potential range 50 – 1400.

Questions

1. What is the differential diagnosis at the time of first admission?
2. Which physiological homeostatic mechanisms are disturbed in this patient?
3. What treatment should be given and what is the prognosis?

Leading Questions

1. (a) Which diseases are suggested by the excessive fluid intake and loss with which the patient presented?
   (b) Is the patient's salt craving related to other signs and symptoms?
   (c) Are there any diseases suggested by your answers to 1.(a) which are more or less likely in view of the patient's symptoms of cramp, vertigo and weakness?
   (d) How do nausea and vomiting fit into the developing clinical picture?

2. (a) There are two basic reasons why the measured concentration of plasma sodium may be low. What are they?
   (b) How does the body detect changes in plasma sodium? Which structures are responsible for it?
   (c) Where is the sodium concentration of the plasma regulated and what mechanisms are involved?
   (d) In what circumstance does the sodium concentration in a random specimen of urine give useful information?
   (e) Which disorders are suggested by the continuing excretion of sodium in the presence of hyponatraemia?
   (f) Is there any evidence to implicate either the control mechanisms or the site(s) of their regulatory action in the genesis of hyponatraemia?
   (g) Water balance is regulated by two mechanisms. What are they? Which structures control it?
   (h) What processes can cause perturbations of the plasma osmolality?
   (i) In what circumstances is urea a good indicator of dehydration and when does it fail?
   (j) What is the significance of the measured urine osmolality in this patient?
   (k) What evidence is there for hypovolaemia and why is it present?
3. (a) What are the objectives in treatment in the short and long term?
   (b) What dietary or other measures are indicated and what are their dangers?
   (c) Can the patient's anaemia be treated?
   (d) What long term treatment is available?

Discussion

The patient presents with a wide spectrum of signs and symptoms of which the most informative are those of increased fluid intake, polyuria with nocturia and polydipsia. With polyuria and polydipsia the diagnostic possibilities include diabetes mellitus or insipidus, chronic renal disease or compulsive water drinking. Salt craving would indicate that the patient has salt loss which needs constant replacement; while the symptoms of cramp, vertigo and weakness suggest that the salt loss is severe enough to cause a reduction in total body sodium and hyponatraemia. Since the patient is vomiting, sodium may be lost from the gastrointestinal tract; however, nausea and vomiting are also symptoms of renal failure (CRF) and the other symptoms including nocturia and polyuria together with the proteinuria lend support to renal loss of sodium being the principal cause.

Routine biochemical tests provide confirmation of the clinical diagnosis of hyponatraemia and renal failure with low plasma sodium, raised plasma urea and reduced creatinine clearance. Normal plasma glucose and the absence of glycosuria eliminate diabetes mellitus as a cause of the biochemical abnormalities. Hypernatraemia would be the expected finding in diabetes insipidus. Psychogenic water drinking may give rise to severe hyponatraemia with fits but other renal function tests with the possible exception of tubular concentrating ability would be normal. Thus CRF seems to be the most likely diagnosis.

Sodium balance in CRF

CRF is caused by a large number of different diseases of which glomerulonephritis, pyelonephritis, polycystic kidney disease and multi-system disorders account for about 70 per cent. Sodium balance is liable to be disturbed in the direction of either hyper-natraemia or hyponatraemia. In the majority of patients with CRF tubular function is able, for a time, to adjust to a reduced glomerular filtration rate, with its potential for sodium retention, by reabsorbing a smaller fraction of the filtered sodium ('glomerular-tubular balance'). Eventually glomerular damage becomes so severe that renal excretion of sodium is inadequate, so leading to hyper-natraemia. In contrast, in those renal diseases in which tubular damage predominates, e.g., pyelonephritis, polycystic kidney disease, nephrocalcinosis and analgesic nephropathy, the patient can present with 'salt losing nephritis' with excessive losses of both salt and water but with a relatively greater loss of sodium. Hyponatraemia is the result. The condition is not confined to active tubular disease; it can occur also in the recovery phase of acute tubular necrosis or after the relief of obstructive uropathy.

Regulation of plasma sodium

Sodium is the chief cation in the extracellular fluid and together with its associated anions accounts for approximately 90 per cent of the osmolality of plasma. The sodium concentration is, therefore, an important factor in the maintenance of plasma osmolality; water balance is the other. Both are closely interrelated and adjusted in view of the need to control the distribution of water between the intercellular, extracellular and intravascular compartments but especially the circulating blood volume. Sodium concentration is maintained by altering renal excretion which is the result of a balance between glomerular filtration and tubular reabsorption. A large quantity of sodium is filtered even when GFR is greatly reduced, e.g., at a GFR of 5ml. $min.^{-1}$ and plasma sodium of 140mmol. ℓ^{-1} approximately 1000 mmol sodium is filtered each day. It follows, therefore, that the control of sodium excretion is almost entirely achieved by altering reabsorption of this filtered sodium. The major fraction of filtered sodium is normally reabsorbed with water in the proximal convoluted tubule. Fine regulation occurs in the distal tubule and collecting ducts under the control of mineralocorticoids (in particular aldosterone), the sympathetic nervous system and a third factor, the, as yet unidentified, natriuretic hormone. The renin-angiotensin-aldosterone mechanism is activated by reduction in renal blood flow resulting from a fall either in blood pressure of blood volume: more sodium and water is reabsorbed leading to restoration of effective blood volume. Angiotensin II also has a vaso-constricting action which raises blood pressure.

Regulation of body water

Water balance is mainly controlled by varying excretion but in addition the thirst mechanism regulates intake. Excretion is controlled by antidiuretic hormone (ADH) which acts on the collecting tubule to increase the permeability of the cells to water so leading to the production of concentrated urine. Two types of receptor modulate ADH secretion. Those found in the anterior hypothalamus are responsive to the osmotic changes brought about by changes in plasma sodium or in other solutes unable to pass through cell membranes and they keep plasma osmolality within a narrow range. It should be noted in this context that urea is a diffusible solute which enters cells rapidly and although it contributes to measured plasma osmolality in CRF, it does not affect the osmotic gradient across the cell membrane of the osmoreceptors. Thus in CRF with hyponatraemia effective plasma osmolality is low, despite the uraemia and consequently the osmoreceptors would tend to reduce ADH secretion in order to raise the osmolality of the plasma. Receptors sensitive to alterations in ECF and plasma volume are found in the left atrium and respond by releasing ADH leading to water retention. Under these circumstances of hypovolaemia the osmoreceptors become less sensitive to hypo-osmolality. On balance, therefore, ADH secretion would increase and so lower the osmolality while increasing the plasma volume.

Clinical assessment of water depletion depends almost entirely on physical examination. The rise in plasma urea, one of the usual biochemical indicators of dehydration, loses its diagnostic value in the presence of renal failure.

Significance of hyponatraemia

Hyponatraemia is a common finding in hospitalized patients; in one series 15 per cent of patients had plasma sodium concentrations of less than 134 mmol. ℓ^{-1}. Understanding the causes and mechanism of hyponatraemia is, therefore, essential if unnecessary treatment is to be prevented in the majority of these patients in whom the finding is of no real significance. Spurious hyponatraemia may result from dilution with fluid of low sodium concentration when taking the blood sample close to the site of an IV infusion. Pseudohyponatraemia is found in patients with greatly increased concentrations of lipid or protein in the plasma for methodological reasons. These macromolecules occupy a significant volume (larger in gross hyperlipaemia or hyperproteinaemia) which is included in the 'plasma volume' measured for the determination of sodium concentration by flame photometry. Such determinations, therefore, underestimate the true sodium concentration in plasma, which may well be correctly controlled by osmoregulation; the resulting apparent hyponatraemia obviously warrants no corrective therapy.

True hyponatraemia can be caused by increases in body water, increased net loss of sodium or changes in distribution of sodium and/or water between the different fluid compartments of the body. In any individual patient more than one factor may be operating. Investigation will involve the following biochemical determinations: plasma urea and electrolytes; plasma osmolality (measured and calculated); urine sodium excretion; creatinine clearance and urine osmolality. Results must be interpreted with full knowledge of the clinical state of the patient. For example, the isolated measurement of urine osmolality as carried out in this patient can be evaluated only if fluid intake and the state of hydration is known and possibly controlled. A normally functioning kidney can produce urine of a very high or low osmolality, with a range of $50 - 1400$ mmol. kg^{-1}, depending on fluid and solute intake. In the same way interpreting the urine excretion of sodium requires the knowledge of the plasma sodium concentration, sodium intake and the degree of hydration. (Treatment with diuretics renders the interpretation of urine sodium almost impossible.) These caveats have not been observed in this patient, neither the sodium nor the water intake being known.

Appropriate *vs* inappropriate ADH secretion

In the presence of hyponatraemia and clinical volume depletion the continuing excretion of urine of high sodium content would indicate renal salt wasting or adrenal insufficiency. The increased plasma urea and serum phosphate together with the normal plasma potassium and markedly reduced creatinine clearance supports the former diagnosis. On the other hand, if the body fluid is normal or increased, the syndrome of inappropriate ADH secretion (SIADH) should be considered. For this diagnosis to be valid, the patient must be in sodium balance, have normal blood pressure, skin turgor and adrenocortical function and produce concentrated urine despite plasma hypo-osmolality. It should be noted that the presence of hypovolaemia excludes SIADH: the condition actually triggers an appropriate secretion of ADH, the response of the osmoreceptors to hypo-osmolality being weak in these circumstances, as described above. A misdiagnosis of SIADH is of crucial importance since treatment usually includes water restriction which is contraindicated in patients with hypovolaemia.

Serum urate has been found to be low in patients with true SIADH and may be a useful investigation in difficult cases. The exact reason for this hypouricaemia is not clear but it appears to be a consequence of increased urate clearance secondary to water expansion; the decrease in serum urate is much greater than one would expect from simple dilution. ADH itself has been shown to reduce urate clearance and is, therefore, not the cause. Serum urate and urate clearance return to normal with fluid restriction. Measurement of ADH in patients with SIADH has produced conflicting results. In those cases associated with malignancy very high ADH concentrations have been found but in other cases ADH has been normal or even low.

Sequelae of CRF

Laboratory data demonstrate a number of other abnormalities associated with CRF. There is retention of phosphate with a concomitant fall in serum calcium which has presumably been largely compensated by secondary hyperparathyroidism. A metabolic acidosis is also present due to a reduced ability to excrete titratable acid and generate ammonia. The patient's haematological indices are not typical of CRF: usually a deficiency of erythropoietin results in a normochromic normocytic anaemia. In severe uraemia red cell half-life is reduced and gastrointestinal bleeding may occur which can superimpose microcytosis and hypochromia due to iron loss. Body iron stores are reduced and this is normally reflected in reduced serum ferritin concentrations.

Aetiology

When a patient first presents with chronic renal failure in adult life it is often very difficult to establish the exact aetiology even if histological examination of the kidney is possible. In the case under consideration the salt losing state suggests certain renal diseases and questions should be asked concerning possible renal infections in childhood and family and analgesic history. Radiology and ultrasound examination may show nephrocalcinosis, cysts or abnormalities of the renal tract.

Therapy

Management of this patient involves attention to sodium and water balance. Oral intake of salt and water should be encouraged but the danger of overloading particularly with water must be emphasized. A reduction of protein intake is necessary to lower blood urea; at the same time it is important to keep calorie intake high with carbohydrate and fat in order to prevent nitrogen loss. Treatment of any bone disease induced by the secondary hyperparathyroidism is effected with vitamin D analogue 1 hydroxy vitamin D or the active metabolite 1,25 dihydroxy vitamin D. The anaemia is often refractory to treatment, although iron deficiency can be corrected and haemolysis reduced by lowering urea. Transfusion occasionally may be required. The prognosis of chronic renal failure is variable, some patients will survive for several years with very low GFRs. However, eventually dialysis or transplantation will become necessary.

Additional Questions

1. How can osmolality be calculated from measurement of major plasma solutes? In what circumstances is the difference between measured and calculated osmolalities useful?
2. Could the patient's hyponatraemia be due to movement of water from the intracellular to the extracellular space?

Further Reading

Flear, C. G. T., Gill, G. V. and Burn, J. (1981). Hyponatraemia Mechanisms and Management. *Lancet* **ii** pp. 26–31.
Harrington, J. T. and Cohen, J. J. (1975). Measurement of Urinary Electrolytes – Indications and Limitations. *New England Journal of Medicine* **293** pp, 1241–1243.

Case 19

Case History

P. T., a 61-year-old store manager, was admitted to hospital for investigation. He had been seeing his GP over the last few months complaining of indigestion and a sensation of fullness in the epigastrium. From time to time he experienced a severe cramp-like pain in the right upper quadrant, radiating to the scapular area, associated with vomiting, especially after a heavy meal. On several occasions he had developed fever, with temperatures up to 38·5 °C, shivering, followed by exacerbation of pain, vomiting, passing of dark urine and pruritus. His bowels were normal. He had lost 2 or 3 lbs over the past 6 months.

Examination

The patient was jaundiced, temperature 38 °C.
AS Tenderness in right subcostal region. Liver not enlarged.
All other systems: no abnormality detected.

Laboratory Investigations

Investigation	Results Day 1	Day 4	Day 10	Day 14	Reference range
Haemoglobin (g/dl)	14·5				13·0–17·0
RBC ($10^{12}. \ell^{-1}$)	5·0				4·2–6·5
WBC ($10^9. \ell^{-1}$)	15	17			4·0–11·0
Serum bilirubin (Total) (μmol. ℓ^{-1})	40	220 (unconjugated 85)	55	35	3–20
Alkaline phosphatase (IU. ℓ^{-1})	150	650	350	95	30–110
Alanine aminotransferase (IU. ℓ^{-1}) (ALT)	40	65	70	75	15–55
Serum albumin (g. ℓ^{-1})	43		42		35–50
Urine bilirubin	+	++	+	0	0
Urine urobilinogen	(+)	0	0	+	(+)
Stools (colour)	normal	clay-colour	normal	normal	
Blood culture	E. coli	E. coli	—	—	

Questions

1. What is the differential diagnosis?
2. What further tests should be done?

eading Questions

. (a) What tentative conclusion can be drawn from the sporadic nature of the pain?
(b) What are the possible sites of origin of a pain in the upper quadrant and which of them are unlikely in this patient?
(c) What do the triad fever, shivering and jaundice suggest?
(d) Which common cause of jaundice can be ruled out by the laboratory tests on day 1?
(e) Is there any indication of hepatocellular damage on day 1?
(f) What is the most likely explanation of the septicaemia?
(g) Which single explanation best fits the laboratory data on day 4?
(h) What do the biochemical changes seen on days 10 and 14 signify?
(i) What is the diagnosis at this time?
(j) What further complications may ensue if treatment is delayed?
(k) What is the composition of gall-stones and in what circumstances are they formed?

2. (a) What is the most urgent laboratory test on day 1?
(b) Which laboratory test would give an indication of a sudden extension of the pathology?
(c) Which further investigation is the safest and liable to be the most revealing?
(d) Which investigation should not be done until after the infection has been eliminated?

Discussion

Here is a patient in the age group at risk from cardiovascular and neoplastic disease, with abdominal pain. The history of symptoms over a few months suggests a chronic condition and the site could be consistent with peptic ulcer, gall-stones and cholecystitis, chronic pancreatitis, angina pectoris, irritable bowel syndrome and carcinoma of the right colon. The absence of diarrhoea rules out irritable bowel syndrome. Angina pectoris would be expected to be relieved by a few minutes' rest and is not particularly associated with meals, which appears to be the case in this patient.

The periodic fever suggests an infection of fluctuating severity. A possible involvement of the liver and biliary tract is indicated by vomiting, dark urine, pruritus, jaundice and subcostal tenderness. In fact, fever, shivering and jaundice constitute the classic triad of Charcot, indicating acute cholangitis.

Laboratory tests on day 1 show a raised serum bilirubin with overflow of the conjugated pigment into the urine. (Unconjugated bilirubin, being water-insoluble and carried by albumin in the plasma, is not excreted in the kidney.) In the absence of anaemia a haemolytic cause of the bilirubinaemia can be ruled out and the differential diagnosis is between hepatocellular and obstructive jaundice. Alkaline phosphatase is raised, but not greatly; however, a serum ALT and albumin concentration within normal limits indicate the absence of generalized parenchymal disease. Thus the information available at this stage favours a partial and intermittent intrahepatic or extrahepatic obstruction. It should be noted here that γ-glutamyl-transferase, widely believed to be a more sensitive indicator than alkaline phosphatase, is of little value in the differential diagnosis of liver disease and has no real advantages over alkaline phosphatase except possibly in paediatrics.

The nature of the infective organisms cultured from the blood suggests that they are of intestinal origin and that they may have been regurgitated from a blocked bile duct.

Increasing obstruction

On day 4, during an attack, the serum bilirubin is much higher and this is reflected in the 2+ urinary pigment. Some of the serum bilirubin is unconjugated which signifies either a partial failure of conjugation or regurgitation of previously conjugated pigment which has been hydrolyzed by deconjugating bacteria in the biliary system.

The ALT is slightly raised but not to a level suggestive of hepatocellular damage (4–40 times the upper normal limit). In contrast, the alkaline phosphatase is several times the upper normal limit which is characteristic of obstruction (*see* Case 9) and tallies with the disappearance of urobilinogen from the urine (since none can be formed in the gut when obstruction is complete) and with the clay-coloured stools. Steatorrhoea may be present at this stage due to the failure of emulsification of fat in the absence of bile salts and possibly to a blockage of the pancreatic duct and consequent lack of lipase.

On days 10 and 14 both serum bilirubin and alkaline phosphatase can be seen to have declined dramatically. Clearly, the obstruction has been partially relieved: less bile pigment and alkaline phosphatase is regurgitated into the blood-stream, urobilinogen reappears in the urine and stercobilin in the faeces.

Pending further investigations, a tentative diagnosis of choledocholithiasis (gall-stone in the common bile duct) with intermittent obstruction can be made. The obstruction is usually partial, the stone acting like a ball valve, sometimes closing the lower end of the bile duct and at other times allowing bile to pass through into the gut. The stagnant bile is readily infected by intestinal bacteria which contribute to the build-up of intraluminal pressure. Eventually this results in reflux of bile into the hepatic venous blood and hence in septicaemia which can be catastrophic if the obstruction is complete and prolonged. The intermittent nature of the blockage is reflected in the fluctuating fever, depth of jaundice and pruritus, the latter being due to the regurgitation of bile salts.

Biliary stasis may be aggravated by inflammatory changes in the ductal mucosa – oedema, thickening and possibly ulceration – which may spread to the intrahepatic bile ducts and, if prolonged, may give rise to cholangitic abscesses and ultimately biliary cirrhosis. When the ampulla of Vater is blocked by stones, bile may be regurgitated along the pancreatic duct and so cause acute or chronic pancreatitis.

Cholesterol stone formation

Gall-stones are of two types: more than 90 per cent have cholesterol as their main component; the remainder consist of bile pigment and occur only in patients with haemolytic disease. The propensity of cholesterol to form stones is attributable to its poor water solubility. In bile it is kept in micellar solution by bile acids and lecithin.

Bile is frequently supersaturated with respect to cholesterol even in normal individuals, but supersaturation is an insufficient, if necessary, precondition for stone formation. It occurs in the hepatocyte rather than the gall baldder, as sampling of bile directly from the liver has shown, and it implies an imbalance between the relative amounts of cholesterol and bile acid. Overproduction of cholesterol in obese subjects on a high calorie diet or inadequate reabsorption of bile acids from the gut may be responsible. Since the enterohepatic circulation normally returns 95 per cent of the excreted bile acids to the liver, any interference with the reabsorption is liable to predispose to gall-stone formation. Conditions such as ileitis, ileal resection or bypass, cystic fibrosis or diarrhoea lead to faecal loss of bile acids which cannot be made good by synthesis *de novo*. Even the temporary interruption of bile acid circulation during the night, when the sphincter of Oddi is closed and the bile flows into the gall bladder, is associated with supersaturation since the nocturnal secretion of cholesterol continues unabated.

Actual precipitation of cholesterol monohydrate from the supersaturated bile depends on the presence or absence, in the gall bladder or bile ducts, of nucleating agents or inhibitors, whose importance may be as great as that of the relative rates of cholesterol or bile acid secretion. Equally crucial is the rate of growth of the incipient stone(s), which may be slow or fast in relation to the frequency of emptying of the gall bladder: biliary stasis clearly favours stone formation.

Other investigations

Other investigations are required for an assessment of the nature and extent of the biliary stasis:

1. After identification of the infecting organisms in the blood, their antibiotic sensitivity must be determined so that appropriate therapy can be rapidly instituted.
2. Determination of serum amylase which may be raised if a blockage of the pancreatic duct has given rise to pancreatitis.
3. Ultrasound imaging can detect even minimal enlargements of the biliary tree due to an obstruction.
4. A plain X-ray to visualize any gall-stones in the gall bladder and bile ducts, bearing in mind that only 10–15 per cent of stones are sufficiently calcified to be radiopaque.

5. Retrograde endoscopic cholangiography which can often reveal a stone but which should not be attempted until after successful antibiotic treatment to avoid spreading the infection up the pancreatic duct.

Additional Questions

1. Is there any indication for determining the prothrombin time before and after vitamin K?
2. Why is an early diagnosis particularly important?

Further Reading

La Morte, W. W., Matolo, N. M., Birkett, D. H. and Williamson Jr., L. F., (1981). Pathogenesis of cholesterol gall-stones, *Surg. Clin. North Amer.*, **61**, pp. 765–773.
Sherlock, S. (1981) *Diseases of the Liver and Biliary system*, pp. 476–496, Blackwell Scientific Publications, Oxford.

Case 20

Case History

David S., aged 11 years, was admitted to the children's hospital with suspected diabetes and ketonuria. He had been well, apart from the usual children's ailments, until about 4 weeks prior to admission when he had a mild respiratory infection. Shortly afterwards he had become aware of polydipsia, especially at night, and polyuria. He had lost weight despite a voracious appetite and he complained of fatigue. The GP was consulted and found glycosuria and ketonuria and referred David to Hospital.

Examination

The patient was on the 75th centile for height, but his weight was below the 25th centile. He appeared mildly dehydrated with dry tongue and loose skinfolds. No other abnormalities were found on examination except for generalized lymphadenopathy and sluggish reflexes.

Laboratory investigations

Investigation	Result	Reference range
Blood glucose (random) (mmol ℓ^{-1})	29	3·4 – 6·7
Plasma urea (mmol ℓ^{-1})	9·2	2·5 – 7·5
Plasma sodium (mmol ℓ^{-1})	143	135 – 146
Plasma potassium (mmol ℓ^{-1})	3·6	3·3 – 5·3
Plasma chloride (mmol ℓ^{-1})	100	98 – 108
Plasma bicarbonate (mmol ℓ^{-1})	18	22 – 26
Urine glucose (mmol ℓ^{-1})	360	negative
Urine ketones	+ +	negative

Questions

1. Would you request any further laboratory tests at this stage?
2. What treatment would you prescribe?
3. What is the likely course of the disease over the next few weeks, months or years and how would this be manifested in laboratory tests? How would treatment have to be adapted?
4. What are the major problems in the treatment of juveniles?

Leading Questions

1. (a) Is the diagnosis unambiguous in the case described?
   (b) Are there any other conditions which give rise to hyper-glycaemia?
   (c) If the patient had come to the doctor's notice 3 weeks earlier, which test might have been appropriate and informative?
2. (a) What is the immediate objective of therapy and how is it achieved?
   (b) How is the therapy in the following few days guided by the biochemical assessment?
3. (a) In which respects does Type I (Insulin Dependent) diabetes IDDM) differ from type II (Non-insulin dependent) Diabetes Mellitus?
   (b) Why is IDDM ultimately not treatable by diet and oral hypo-glycaemics?
   (c) Does the endogenous production of insulin in IDDM vary over the course of the disease?
   (d) What is C-peptide? How does its determination help in assessing the diabetic state?
4. (a) In the short term, which two hazards accompany therapy?
   (b) How can they be prevented by home monitoring? What are the shortcomings of these methods?
   (c) Is there a means of obtaining an overall picture of exposure of cells to high glucose concentrations?

Discussion

A random blood glucose in excess of 11 mmol ℓ^{-1} is strongly suggestive of diabetes, especially if ketone bodies are present in the urine. The presentation with polydipsia, polyuria, weight loss and fatigue over a 3–4 week period is typical of Type 1 (Insulin dependent) diabetes (IDDM) with its precipitous loss of B-cell function. Other causes must be investigated in cases of milder hyperglycaemia since acute illness, stress, some liver diseases, uraemia, or excessive secretion of growth hormone, thyroxine, cortisone and adrenaline all lower glucose tolerance. Under these circumstances a glucose tolerance test may be useful; in the present case it is not necessary.

Management

Treatment is initially with insulin, often 0·5U/kg/day, by continuous IV infusion to bring the blood glucose down quickly to normal levels and to eliminate the ketonaemia. In most cases the dose can be substantially reduced in the course of 2–3 weeks, the degree of glucosuria being a guide to insulin administration. In some cases, after initial treatment, the requirement for insulin falls so that little or none needs to be given in conjunction with dietary measures. This 'honeymoon' period can last from a few weeks to some months at most, after which insulin requirements increase until total dependence on exogenous hormone supervenes.

As a consequence of the diuresis associated with glucosuria the patient will have lost both water and electrolytes, particularly potassium. In the conscious patient this can be quickly replaced orally but in coma the intravenous route is necessary. Although the plasma potassium may be within the normal range owing to a shift of the ion out of the cells, the total body potassium is always low and replacement is essential.

Aetiology

IDDM, misleadingly referred to as juvenile onset diabetes, differs from Type II (non-insulin dependent) diabetes in several ways which reflect the different aetiologies of the conditions. It is associated with the HLA antigens which are known to be related to the immune response genes. Thus an immunological mechanism may be expected to be an important part of the aetiology. Newly diagosed patients' sera can often, but not always, be shown to contain antibodies to B-cells; the failure to demonstrate their presence in some cases may turn out to be methodological. Round-cell infiltration of the endocrine pancreas characterizes the pathology of the disease. Although IDDM is a heterogeneous disorder, in most cases it seems to result from autoimmune destruction of the B-cells, triggered by a virus infection. Thus the hereditary element, though undoubted, is not strong, as witness the relatively low (40 per cent) concordance rates in identical twins, and is thought to be a propensity to respond to virus, especially coxsackie, by an autoimmune reaction. The cell-mediated autoimmunity and cytotoxic reactions are believed to contribute to the cellular destruction in the acute phase and often not more than 10 per cent of the B-cell population remains intact after the initial assault.

It has been suggested that early vigorous control of the diabetes might somehow blunt the autoimmune attack and enable the remaining B-cells to continue functioning for some time, so accounting for the remission which is a common feature of IDDM. The remission is usually only partial and rarely complete and can last for weeks or months, but so far there is no convincing evidence that it can be prolonged by meticulous control of the blood glucose. Its occurrence has no prognostic value. After 6–18 months of therapy and often after another viral infection insulin requirements begin to rise inexorably towards total dependence.

Evidence for endogenous secretion of insulin during remission comes from the determination of C-peptide in patients' plasma. C-peptide is the connecting peptide between the A and B chains or proinsulin. It is formed in equimolar amounts with insulin by hydrolysis of the precursor protein within the storage granules and simultaneously released into the blood stream. Unlike insulin, the C-peptide has no biological activity and therefore its amino acid sequence has not been conserved in the course of evolution; there is thus a considerable interspecies variation. The radioimmunological assay of human insulin in the presence of exogenous porcine or bovine insulin is not possible due to cross-reaction of the almost identical insulin molecules with the antibody. Furthermore, after treatment with exogenous insulin, anti-insulin antibodies are produced which also interfere with radioimmunoassay. Specific C-peptide assay, on the other hand, is possible even in the presence of C-peptide or proinsulin from other species. Thus C-peptide can be used to study residual endogenous secretion in the early stages of IDDM, including the remission phase.

With the destruction of the remaining B-cells exogenous insulin becomes essential and hence dietary or oral drug therapy is of no avail in IDDM in the long run. In this respect also the disease differs radically from Type II diabetes.

Metabolic derangements

The glucose intolerance of IDDM is a result of both under-utilization of glucose in the peripheral tissues and overproduction by gluconeogenesis in the liver. Alanine and, indirectly, branched chain amino acids provide the carbon skeleton for glucose synthesis, the nitrogen being excreted as urea. Lipid metabolism, too, is affected. The concentrations of all lipid fractions in the serum are usually raised, including triglyceride, cholesterol and free fatty acids, with long-term implications for the development of atheromatous plaques. An acceleration of lipolysis in the fat depots not only elevates the plasma FFA, sometimes to double the normal concentration, but the liver cells become loaded with fat droplets. At the same time alterations in hepatic metabolism, especially a greatly enhanced transfer of fatty acids to the mitochondria, increase β-oxidation of fatty acids and hence production of acetylCoA.

The rate of this process is such as to exceed the capacity of the citric acid cycle to oxidize acetylCoA which therefore accumulates and condenses to acetoacetate and so leads to formation of acetone and β-hydroxybutyrate. The resulting ketonaemia is further exacerbated by a defective metabolism of ketone bodies in muscle, possibly as a result of inadequate activity of hydroxybutyrate dehydrogenase in the absence of insulin. Thus ketosis can be seen to be the consequence of three distinct biochemical changes triggered by lack of insulin: increased lipolysis in adipose tissue, stimulation of fatty acid oxidation in the liver and reduced ability of the muscle to metabolize ketone bodies. The mechanism of ketogenesis in starvation is qualitatively the same but the metabolic derangements are less severe.

Ketoacidosis and hypoglycaemia are the result of under- and overtreatment of the juvenile diabetic patient. Since both dietary intake and exercise greatly influence glucose metabolism and hence insulin requirement, the difficulty of achieving control, particularly in a child, will be appreciated. It is reflected in frequent swings between hyperglycaemia and hypoglycaemia. The latter, if extreme, is associated with seizures or coma which may give rise to permanent EEG abnormalities. Hyperglycaemia carries the risk of ketoacidosis and eventually of neuropathy, currently believed to be due to formation of sorbitol by interaction of glucose with NADP.

This reaction, which takes place only at high glucose concentrations, has two consequences: the cell accumulates sorbitol which cannot pass through the membrane and thus causes osmotic swelling, and, at the same time, there develops a deficiency of NADP.

While the precise connection of microvascular disease with the metabolic derangements of inadequately controlled diabetes remains unclear, normalization of blood glucose is the only potential prophylactic measure available at this time.

Control of glucose

On a day-to-day basis urine glucose estimation, done at home, gives a moderately satisfactory picture of the adequacy of treatment. For a variety of reasons, which includes variation of renal thresholds, the correspondence between blood and urine levels is not good. Home monitoring of blood glucose is a more reliable method of assessment, albeit unpopular with small children, although the spring-loaded blood letting lance has made the method of obtaining blood more acceptable. If blood glucose levels are 13·3 mmol ℓ^{-1} (240mg/dl) or greater, urine ketones should be checked and if these are moderate or large, supplementary insulin must be given.

One problem associated with blood glucose monitoring is that the frequency and duration of the hypoglycaemic and hyperglycaemic episodes between sampling remain largely unknown. By comparison, the ability of the healthy pancreatic B cell to fulfill this function and act accordingly, cannot as yet be approached, let alone equalled.

Recently it was discovered that exposure of red cells to high glucose concentrations leads to glucosylation of haemoglobin A to HbA_{1c}. The free amino group of the β-chain reacts with glucose to form first a Schiff's base and then a ketoamine:

Glucose   β-chain   Schiff's base   Ketoamine

The speed of this non-enzymatic glucosylation depends critically on the glucose concentration within the red cell and the product of the reaction, which can readily be measured, furnishes an integrated record of the total exposure of the patient's circulating cells to high glucose concentrations throughout their life-span. Thus a regular determination of HbA_{1c} should be a valuable guide to the overall control of glucose metabolism and may, perhaps, prevent some of the complications of diabetes.

Additional Questions

1. What are the biochemical and clinical sequelae of untreated ketoacidosis?
2. What is the long-term prognosis of Type I diabetes?

Further Reading

Brouhard, B. H. (1983), Control and monitoring for the child with insulin dependent diabetes mellitus, *Am. J. Dis. Child*, **137**, pp. 787–792.

Keen, H. and Ng Tang Fui, S. (1982), The definition and classification of diabetes mellitus, *Clinics in Endocrinology and Metabolism*, (1982), **11** (2), pp. 275–305.

Index